The

Getting

Rodger Charlton

GP Principal
Trainer and Tutor
Solihull, West Midlands
and
Senior Lecturer
The Medical School
University of Warwick

Radcliffe Publishing
Oxford • Seattle

Radcliffe Publishing Ltd
18 Marcham Road
Abingdon
Oxon OX14 1AA
United Kingdom

www.radcliffe-oxford.com
Electronic catalogue and worldwide online ordering facility.

British Library Cataloguing in Publication Data

A catalogue record for this book is available from the British Library.

ISBN 1 85775 632 0

Typeset by Acorn Bookwork Ltd, Salisbury, Wiltshire
Printed and bound by TJ International Ltd, Padstow, Cornwall

Contents

About the author

Rodger Charlton BA MB ChB MPhil MD FRCGP FRNZCGP DFFP FSOMW qualified from Birmingham in 1983. During vocational training in Nottingham he completed an MPhil thesis in medical ethics. Shortly afterwards he became a GP principal in Derby in a five-doctor partnership and part-time lecturer in general practice at Nottingham University. In 1991–92, he was a visiting fellow at the Department of General Practice, University of Otago Medical School, New Zealand, researching into the perceived needs of undergraduates in palliative medicine education. This formed the basis of his MD thesis. He also worked as a GP in New Zealand gaining his MRNZCGP in 1992.

In 1994 he was appointed as a senior lecturer in primary healthcare at the Postgraduate School of Medicine, Keele University, and in 1995 he took over a single-handed general practice in Hampton-in-Arden, close to the Warwickshire border. In 1997 he became a GP trainer and in 1998 he became editor of the Royal College of General Practitioners (RCGP) *Members' Reference Book* (MRB) for two years. He is now the editor of RCGP publications excluding the journal and MRB which is now produced quarterly as the TNG (*The New Generalist*).

His research interests and published papers are in palliative care, bereavement and meningococcal disease, but there is a strong focus on research in education and professional development in primary care. In September 2000 he was appointed as senior lecturer in continuing professional development at Warwick University and in January 2003 he became the Director of GP Undergraduate Medical Education at Warwick Medical School. He received the John Fry Award of the RCGP in April 2001 for being a GP who has 'promoted the discipline of general practice through research and publishing as a practising GP'.

In November 2003 he was awarded a fellowship of the Society of Medical Writers (SOMW) of which he became the chairman in April 2004. He maintains an interest in postgraduate education by being a GP and primary care trust (PCT) tutor and helping GPs move through the recent changes in relation to the Postgraduate Education Allowance (PGEA), personal development plans (PDPs) and appraisal. He has now become a GP Appraiser.

Rodger has been a GP principal for 16 years and during this time has acquired knowledge in the day-to-day running of a GP practice. During his five years as a solo practitioner until he went into partnership in September 2000, he had to get to grips with practice management and how a GP and GP practice gets paid and the many associated issues. This has remained an interest since then particularly with the advent of the new GP contract (nGMS contract, also called GMS II). As well as being an academic GP he remains a practical 'hands on' GP both in patient care and the running of a practice with his GP partner, Ryan Prince.

To all general practitioners that this text may be a help to them
as they cope with further change.

Introduction

In June 2003, GPs (family doctors) in the UK overwhelmingly (80%) supported a new contract which has been hailed by some as the biggest change in their employment terms since the NHS was founded in 1948. As well as being paid for 'essential' services which are the 'core' activity of a GP's daily work, GPs would be paid for quality of care in relation to chronic disease and the organisation of care. In addition, it has been recognised that this new contract could enable GPs to provide and be paid for 'enhanced services' traditionally confined to hospitals and so formalise the concept of GPs with Special Interests (GPswSIs).

Although there may be some differences in process in each of the four countries of the UK, the principles of the new contract apply to all. GP practices have been busy preparing for 1 April 2004. Across the four countries of the UK, nearly 100% of practices signed up to the contract, with only eight default contracts in England and none in the other three countries.

One of the problems with the 'new contract' is that there are still a lot of unknowns and ongoing changes, particularly in interpretation and putting the theoretical proposals into practice. I recently received an email from a colleague in France who told me how she kept hearing about the NHS's 'new GP contract', but could not find a simple description of what it was. I was asked if I could tell her in a few words what it was all about, what were the main changes and how it differed from the 1990 contract. As I grappled with this question I was stimulated to answer the question and so write this book and in particular to detail its implications financially to GPs.

Why did the new contract come about?

There are many possible reasons, but one that politicians often quote is that an increase in pay and the ability to opt out of out-of-hours care would stop GPs leaving the profession. In addition, it would help to recruit newly qualified GPs to take up the increasing number of vacancies and encourage junior doctors to consider general practice as a career. The previous health secretary, Alan Milburn, delegated the responsibility for negotiating the new contract to the NHS Confederation, the representative body for health service managers, because government talks through the Department of Health with the British Medical Association (BMA) reached a deadlock over nearly a three-year period. The General Practitioners Committee (GPC) of the BMA, the professional body for all UK doctors, has represented and continues to represent GPs in the negotiations.

Which GPs will the contract affect?

The new contract (GMS2) covers the 36 000 GPs who work under the General Medical Services (GMS1) contract and the approximately 25% of GPs who work under the Personal Medical Services (PMS) scheme. However, the implications are different for PMS practices as they have contracts negotiated locally with commissioning health bodies such as primary care trusts (PCTs). Nevertheless there is likely to be considerable convergence with GMS2 practices, particularly in terms of quality targets.

It has been said that the new contract will succeed or fail depending on the future partnerships of GPs, GP practices and primary care organisations (PCOs) – PCTs in England and Health Boards in Scotland.

Patients

The government and negotiators hope that patient care will improve as a result. This is unknown because a pivotal change will be that patients will no longer be registered with an individual GP, but a GP practice. Patients are likely to see a greater range of primary care practitioners and not just a general practitioner. This could be a healthcare assistant, a practice nurse, a nurse practitioner, one of many other healthcare practitioners or a general practitioner. Some have argued that this could be the end of the traditional doctor–patient relationship, continuity of care and the personal doctor. Furthermore, as many GPs opt out of out-of-hours care as a result of the new contract, this will further fragment continuity of care.

What will happen to the term, 'GP principal'?

If GPs are no longer responsible for individually registered patients, but the practice is, what will happen to the concept of a GP principal? Will GPs become consultants in primary care? GP practices may choose to just provide essential care for patients who are acutely or chronically sick, or offer a wider range of services, such as contraception, vaccination, minor surgery, and the management of more complex medical conditions such as multiple sclerosis or epilepsy. It is anticipated that quality of care through a national framework of standards (quality indicators) will be an important focus for GP practices. GPs (principals and non-principals) have been transferred from the supplementary lists of PCOs to lists of 'Medical Performers'. (Any doctor who wishes to perform General Medical Services or Personal Medical Services will have to be included in a PCO Medical Performers list from 1 April 2004.) The terms 'principal' and 'non-principal' are being used less frequently and all are GPs whether that is as partners, salaried doctors or working on a sessional/locum basis. However, in view of readers' familiarity with and the transition in the use of this terminology, the term 'GP principal' is still used during this book.

The role of PCOs

The new contract provides increased scope for collaborative working between practices working in the desired 'clusters' of the new contract, across primary care, as well as with secondary care and social services. But what if GPs decide to opt out of providing 24-hour care, immunisations, contraceptive care or chronic disease management? PCOs will take on the responsibility and commissioning costs for providing alternative providers and instead of much of a patient's care being available in a single practice, they may have to travel to different practices for different services.

The future of primary care

Ultimately this has the potential to fragment primary care and its co-ordination under the original gatekeeper – the GP. In an attempt to increase patient choice, patients may be able to register with more than one practice. This may be required, for example, as the place they live may be very far away from where they work. Quality of care may be compromised as the necessary patient records may not be available in the absence of a universally shared patient-held NHS electronic record. However, concurrent information technology (IT) changes predicted in the NHS may overcome this difficulty.

Payments

This book does not attempt to address the pros and cons of the new contract, but rather how to continue quality of patient care and survive financially under the many logistical unknowns of the new contract. Politicians are of the opinion that payment for quality services by demonstrating evidence of achieving defined indicators and providing enhanced services should encourage the provision of a wider range of services within primary care. It is thought that most GPs' NHS income will rise over the next three years, but the amount will be substantially less than the 50% pay rise mooted when the concept of the new contract was launched in February 2003.

Those practices who provide a wider range of services and meet defined high standards should see a considerable rise in profits. This book aims to instruct GPs and practice managers how to achieve this rise.

Practical points

Throughout the book will be sections provided entitled, 'Practical points', which will emphasise these issues and so alert GPs and practice managers to areas that relate to practice income and thus where practice performance can be improved.

Sources for the book

This book is based on information gained from the following sources:

- *New GMS Contract 2003: Investing in General Practice*. BMA Publication.
- *New GMS Contract 2003: Investing in General Practice. Supporting Documentation*. BMA Publication.
- Lilley R (2003) *The New GP Contract: how to make the most of it*. Radcliffe Medical Press, Oxford.
- Spooner A (2004) *Quality in the New GP Contract*. Radcliffe Medical Press, Oxford.
- Various websites including the BMA website: www.bma.org.uk.
- *British Medical Journal*.

- Commentaries from the medical press including *Pulse, Doctor, General Practitioner, Registrar Update*, Department of Health's (DoH) *GP Bulletin, MedEconomics, Guidelines in Practice* and associated supplements.
- Mailings from the author's local PCT, Solihull, West Midlands.
- The 'LMC Live' website: www.lmclive.co.uk.

Interpretation

The writing of this book and in particular the content has provided a considerable challenge to the author. This is for several reasons and one that has posed the most difficulty has been the initial commentary on the new contract and then further development on different aspects of the new contract. A great amount of material has been read in an attempt to understand the many available sources. Interpretations have been made to make the subject digestible and readable. Although reference has been made to specific documents, the most helpful information to interpret these lengthy documents has come from professional magazines including *Doctor, GP* and *Pulse* and also Internet searches under subject headings. There was very little information provided in peer-reviewed medical journals that the author was able to use to guide the content of this book.

In relation to payments, local variations and different regulations for each of the four countries of the UK, these interpretations *may not be absolute*. It is therefore strongly recommended that if the reader is in doubt they should seek further advice as detailed below.

Future changes

For all of us the new contract is a new area and a huge change from the 1990 GP contract. Furthermore, each individual GP practice has received an individual version of the new contract and so there are differences in localities as well as the four countries of the UK.

After publication

When this book goes into print, further developments, revisions and interpretations of aspects of the new contract will be made and the reader should bear this in mind. Similarly, this book does not purport to be an absolute authority or tablet of stone in relation to the new contract; some interpretations by the author may be open to criticism and similarly there may be some errors.

Further information

It is suggested that when a reader has a query or concern about any issue raised in this book and how it applies to their practice, they should seek clarification from their local PCO in the first instance. If they are unhappy with the advice provided by the PCO, then they should refer to the BMA's publications detailed previously or their website for the very latest information regarding the new contract and associated negotiations which can change quickly as the new contract is implemented. Alternatively, one can seek advice from the BMA, if they are a BMA member. This may be by telephone or by email and failing this a Local Medical Committee (LMC) representative may also be able to give practical and helpful advice.

Having made this statement, it is hoped that this book will be both a useful guide to a complex and very different contract to the previous 1990 GP contract and so be a useful source of reference as one seeks a way through the nGMS contract maze.

Role of the GPC of the BMA

In the BMA *Contract News* (April 2004), Dr John Chisholm, Chairman of the GPC, writes, '*The contract is not perfect and we are by no means complacent*'. He goes on to say, '*The contract is an evolving contract and its development is an ongoing process.*' He emphasises how the GPC will continue to work on the problems and concerns that arise as a result of the implementation of the new contract and as progress and developments occur that these will be posted on their website: www.bma.org.uk/gp contract.

Book as a resource

It is hoped that the book is a valuable resource in a contract that has been thrust on busy GPs who have yet another change to cope with as they try and meet the needs of their patients and practices in many different community settings.

Rodger Charlton
November 2004

CHAPTER 1

Getting paid under the 1990 contract

Before a doctor enters general practice, they will be accustomed to receiving a salary and a payslip detailing deductions for tax and national insurance. This is referred to as the PAYE (Pay-As-You-Earn) method of income tax collection. However, most GPs are self-employed, although salaried GP posts are becoming more common. So, if you start as a GP principal it takes quite an adjustment to receiving a cheque of differing amounts each month according to the profits of the practice which is a small 'business'. The cheque is a gross payment and it is advisable to save 40% in a high interest savings account for a tax bill which is in arrears and also for national insurance payments. The local PCO or Health Board deducts a proportion of your payments as superannuation and so a monthly contribution towards your eventual pension.

What it means to be self-employed

GPs have always been self-employed practitioners, who mix their subcontracted work from the NHS with a small amount of private practice. When the NHS was set up in 1948 GPs kept their independence but agreed to register all patients and provide 24-hour care for them in return for contracted payments. In keeping with the ethos of the NHS, this established universal access to GPs for the first time in the UK. This chapter describes how GPs were paid on the basis, e.g., of the number of patients registered in their name and other payments for defined services until the advent of the 'new contract' of 1 April 2004. It is important to be conversant with the latest version of this, the '1990 contract', in order to understand the financial workings, the origins of payments and implications for the new contract. Many of the principles of being self-employed also apply to this new contract. This chapter is therefore devoted to the derivation of payments under the previous 1990 GP contract.

Gross payments

When a GP receives their first payment it seems a large amount when there have been no deductions and it is tempting to feel rich and spend a lot. However, it is important to start saving for the tax bill, which may be 12 months in coming, as late payment or taking out a loan results in high interest payments. In order to try and reduce the tax bill, GPs are diligent about keeping receipts as some of their business expenses can be put against the tax bill, e.g., car, telephone and equipment bills. The end of each tax year is usually the beginning of April. This is when a GP starts to complete their tax return form and calculate their tax bill (tax liability). It is also important to employ the services of an accountant (whose fees are tax deductible) to make these calculations. One's first impression might be that this is a lot of hassle, but financially there are benefits to being an independent contractor or self-employed. It also means that you are an employer as opposed to being employed and wholly and exclusive business expenses can legitimately reduce the tax bill.

How did GPs get paid under the 1990 contract?

In essence there were and still are two sources; General Medical Services (GMS) and Personal Medical Services (PMS) in addition to private fees. GMS and PMS payments are for providing NHS services to patients registered with individual GPs of the practice partnership. Private fees can be for seeing patients who wish to be seen privately, although this is relatively rare these days. Private fees are more commonly received for completing reports for insurance companies or solicitors and are not part of a GP's NHS service. In addition, GPs may charge for private sick notes, completing a holiday cancellation form, conducting a pre-employment medical or completing a cremation certificate. Also, some GPs act as occupational health physicians for local firms or as school medical officers to private schools. All these activities are sources of private income and could contribute up to 10% or more of a GP's income before they could affect cost or notional rent reimbursement on GP premises.

General Medical Services (GMS)

These were divided into three main areas:

- basic practice allowance and patient registration fees
- target payments
- item of service payments.

Full-time GPs received a basic practice allowance (BPA) for 1200 or more patients registered with them. If they had less than 1200 patients then the BPA was proportionately less. However, in addition to the BPA, the more patients that were registered with a GP, the greater the income through capitation fees. This was a set annual payment for providing care for patients 24 hours a day, 365 days a year. This payment was greater for patients over the ages of 65 and 75. However, with more patients came a greater workload and there was a ceiling number of registered patients after which there were no additional payments.

Target payments were for providing cervical cytology services to women between the ages of 25 and 64. Similarly, there were target payments for providing defined childhood vaccinations to infants and boosters to preschool children. For both groups there were lower and higher targets to achieve a lower and higher payment. In the case of cervical cytology 80% of women within the above age group had to have had a cervical smear in the preceding five years to achieve a higher payment and the only people exempt were those who had had a hysterectomy (lower target = 50%). In the case of vaccinations the target was 90% to achieve a higher payment (lower target = 70%). In both groups patients who chose not to have a smear or have their child vaccinated would still count towards the target payment. Ways of exempting patients in the new contract will be discussed in a later chapter.

Item of service fees could be claimed for providing the following services:

- contraception advice
- inserting an intra-uterine device (IUD)
- administering certain vaccines, e.g., tetanus
- new patient registration health checks
- minor surgery and child health surveillance
- seeing temporary residents
- performing a night visit (for calls received and completed between the hours of 10pm and 8am)
- maternity care
- arresting a dental haemorrhage
- other areas to be listed in the next chapter where they form part of the Global Sum of the new contract.

Doctors who dispense vaccines and injectables or medication in rural areas could and still can attract certain fees through the Prescription Pricing Authority (PPA).

It can be seen from this information that a lot of data needed to be stored either manually or (more usually) on computer so that the necessary individual claims could be made. The new GP contract should reduce this clerical activity through the payment of a 'Global Sum', which is discussed in the next chapter. This reduction in clerical activity has already been achieved for PMS practices where income is based on the last GMS claims and associated uplifts with inflation and pay reviews and changes with a practice list size. Most claims were made in arrears and they could be claimed manually or through computer links with the local PCO or Health Board. A practice manager would play a vital role in the smooth running of this business side of a GP practice.

Other GMS income

For attending 30 hours per year of approved postgraduate educational activity in the three designated areas of health promotion, disease management and service management a fee of almost £3 000 could be claimed each year. This was paid quarterly upon production of certification of attendance and was called the Postgraduate Education Allowance (PGEA).

There were practice activities for which GPs received partial or full reimbursement. For example, for employed staff whose employment is approved and fell within the agreed staff budget, a reimbursement of 70% was usual. Reimbursement was available for the salary of a GP registrar as well as the payment of a small training grant and this will continue under the new contract. Payments for GPs under the 'GP retainer' scheme payments should also continue.

Partial reimbursement may also have been available for computer expenses, such as hardware and software and especially upgrades which will be a particular feature of the new contract. The changes regarding funding of IT will be discussed in a later chapter, but do not form part of what is called the 'Global Sum'.

Payments were also available for health promotion, chronic disease management – e.g., in diabetes and asthma – and locally defined quality initiatives.

One further incentive for new GPs joining a practice was the 'golden hello' scheme of a one-off payment of usually £5000. GPs will need to enquire of local PCOs whether this scheme will continue under the new contract.

Personal Medical Services (PMS)

PMS is very similar to GMS and many practices have converted to PMS subject to agreement with the local PCT. In PMS a budget is estimated on the basis of the previous year's GMS claim and altered according to patient list size. This avoided all the clerical work associated with making individual claims for the above. In addition, it was possible to negotiate 'PMS with growth' and so the creation of salaried nurse and GP posts to undertake new and locally agreed work for the practice in conjunction with the local PCO. The changes to PMS as a result of the new contract are discussed in depth in Chapter 8.

Payments relating to premises

There should initially be no change in the way that premises-related claims and reimbursements are dealt with under the new contract for:

- cost rent and notional rent payments
- hazardous waste
- rates.

General practice as a 'business'

Being a GP involves knowledge of medicine and developing skills in running a business. Usually, each partner in a practice looks after one area of practice income in liaison with the practice manager. It need not be a burden or daunting if it is well organised and efficient and a practice manager can undertake much of the work. Great satisfaction can be gained from achieving quality patient care and in the same way maximising income to which a GP is entitled. It allows for a degree of independence which employed hospital doctors do not have unless they are involved in private practice.

Why tell you all this?

First, it is to understand how the financial origins of the new contract have come about as it is from these figures that the Global Sum of the new contract (discussed in the next chapter) originates. Second, it is to appreciate that there are elements of the 1990 GMS contract that should in the author's interpretation continue as they are paid mainly three months in arrears for work undertaken prior to 1 April 2004. This is detailed in the Appendix. Individual practices will need to discuss and negotiate such potential claims with their local PCO. If a practice is in doubt they should seek advice from their LMC or the GPC of the BMA.

Practical point

Income from the '1990 contract' should not stop on 1 April 2004. Some of it should continue as many of the payments are in arrears and practice managers should ensure that these continue to be paid or have been settled by 1 April 2004. Under the 1990 GMS contract the old regulations allowed for claims to be submitted for up to six years. However, the limit for submitting these claims may be reduced to six months at a PCO's discretion.

CHAPTER 2

The Global Sum

The last chapter on the 1990 contract may at first glance have appeared to be superfluous to this book, but when one tries to fathom out how the 'global sum' has come into being, its relevance should be apparent.

Calculating the Global Sum

Each practice will have a 'Global Sum' (GS) calculated using a formula called the 'Carr-Hill formula' and its associated adjustments based on their list size on 1 April 2004 and the payments they received in the preceding 12 months under the 1990 GP contract for the following.

Fees and allowances per GP:

- basic practice allowance (BPA)
- capitation fees
- out-of-hours payments
- deprivation payments
- Postgraduate Education Allowance (PGEA) and appraisal
- staff reimbursements and employer's superannuation
- health promotion payments (excluding chronic disease management).

Fees per patient:

- new patient registration health checks
- temporary residents
- rural practice payments
- maternity services (excluding intrapartum care)
- night visit fees
- emergency and immediately necessary treatment fees
- arrest of dental haemorrhage
- contraceptive services (FP1001, but not intra-uterine contraceptive device (IUCD) insertion fees)
- adult immunisations (e.g., tetanus boosters)
- child health surveillance
- sessional payments for expected minor surgery
- cervical cytology target payments.

Other fees that should be subsumed into the Global Sum for rural practices are:

- inducement payments
- anaesthetic administration fees.

Disappearance of the 'Red Book' and appearance of the 'Blue Book(s)'

The Global Sum will be the key funding stream for practices as part of their financial allocations. The new Statement of Financial Entitlement (SFE) will replace the old 'Red Book' and so the Statement of Financial Fees and Allowances (SFA) of the 1990 GP contract. There are many similarities between the two books, but whereas the 'Red Book' applied to GP principals, this new SFE applies to the 'contractor' – the practice. Similarly, as the 'Red Book' applied to SFA, the new SFE applies to all doctors working in the practice, whether partners or salaried, e.g., GP retainers.

Practical point
Practices should check the patient numbers that their PCO has used to calculate the Global Sum and that it is the list size on 31 March 2004.

The Global Sum represents practice income and not individual GP income as under the previous 1990 GP contract.

Practical point
The practice is paid as the 'contractor', not the individual GPs in the practice as under the 1990 contract. The Global Sum is calculated quarterly and paid monthly by PCOs.

All the details of the new contract appear in the following two publications:

- BMA Publication, *New GMS Contract 2003: Investing in General Practice*.
- BMA Publication, *New GMS Contract 2003: Investing in General Practice. Supporting Documentation*.

As these are blue in colour, the term 'Blue Book' or 'Blue Books' have been used by some authors.

An arrangement between a practice and a PCO, not the individual GPs

Fees and allowances payments per GP under the 'Red Book' will go, as will applications for new partners and an associated basic practice allowance. The Global Sum will based on the number of patients registered at a practice.

It might be asked who the contract will be between as it will no longer be between individual GPs in a practice and a local PCO. The answer is that the contract will be between a practice and a PCO. The following differences are also important.

- All partners in a practice will be in a contract with the PCO.
- The GPs need not be partners, e.g., they could be employees of the partnership.
- Not all partners need be GPs, e.g., they could be nurses or the practice manager.

The Carr-Hill formula

One of the great difficulties about the new contract is finding information about it and how the detail in relation to the content and payments came into being. This posed a particular problem when writing this book as the author sought to find out explanations. One immediate conundrum was finding what the Carr-Hill formula was and how this has been used to calculate the Global Sum and take into account the payments GPs received in the preceding 12 months under the 1990 GP contract.

Professor Roy Carr-Hill is an economy researcher in the Centre for Health Economics at the University of York. The detail of the Carr-Hill formula is complex and a document that refers to it on the Department of Health website, 'Global Sum Allocation Formula', can be referred to when reading this chapter (www.dh.gov.uk). This was published on 15 March 2004 and supplements the February 2003 publication, 'Investing in General Practice'.

The Carr-Hill resource allocation formula for the new GMS contract includes adjustments based on the following components:

- the age and sex structure of the population, including patients in nursing and residential homes
- the additional needs of the population, relating to morbidity and mortality
- list turnover
- the unavoidable costs of delivering services to the population, including a staff market forces factor and rurality.

Although the Carr-Hill formula was developed in York, the Global Sum is calculated using the National Health Applications and Infrastructure Services (NHAIS) Exeter System, which is yet another acronym for the reader to digest. The NHAIS Exeter System is a software suite used by all PCOs in England and Wales for the administration of cancer screening call/recall programmes and to deal with patient registration and contractor payments. It includes details of each patient's age, sex, postcode and GP.

The NHS Information Authority extracts data from each of the 87 NHAIS Exeter Systems in England and Wales and forwards them to the Centre for Health Economics at York University where they are aggregated into a notional data set referred to as the Attribution Data Set (ADS). The ADS is used to:

- calculate practice populations
- take into account variables as detailed above in particular areas and the impact of these differences to practice populations.

The terminology used in the Department of Health publication, 'Global Sum Allocation Formula', from which this excerpt is derived, is very complex and the reader who wishes to see the document for themselves should go to the www.dh.gov.uk website.

Adjustments using the Carr-Hill formula

The age–sex adjustment takes into account practice populations where there are different potential workloads as a result of the number of patients registered with a practice who are very young or elderly. This is similar to the capitation-based system of the 1990 contract which took into account the three decades of life after the age of 65 years, by an increase in the capitation fee. This should also take into account the more likely place of consultation: for example, in the practice or during a home visit. Similarly, there is an adjustment to take into account patients in nursing and residential homes.

In order to take into account the needs of an individual area (referred to as a 'ward'), and so morbidity and mortality, an adjustment will be made. Again there are similarities with the 1990 contract and payment of deprivation fees. Similarly, the location of a practice is taken into account regarding the costs to employ staff and the population density. The latter again reflects the 1990 contract where rural practice payments could be claimed. There is also a London adjustment.

When the Global Sum is calculated, of which the Carr-Hill formula is a part of the process, a scaling process is made for each adjustment, referred to as 'normalisation'. This is to ensure that there is equal impact for each adjustment. Once a 'practice weighted population' has been calculated after this normalisation, the weighted population is multiplied by £50 to derive the Global Sum. In the case of practices in one of the five London strategic health authorities (SHAs) the unweighted practice population is first multiplied by £2.18.

The adjustment for the turnover of a practice list will also take into account the additional workload generated by patients in their first year of registration with the practice. The Global Sum will also be adjusted with increases or decreases in the practice list size after the baseline period used to make the calculation on 1 April 2004. Again there are similarities with the 1990 contract and payment of new patient registration health check fees.

To calculate a practice entitlement under the Global Sum, the practice weighting is multiplied by the number of patients registered with the practice. An average UK practice, with an average practice weighting, will receive an average of £50 per patient in 2004/05 which will rise to £51 the following year. Global Sum figures are calculated quarterly to reflect changing practice circumstances and will be paid monthly by PCOs.

Like many parts of the new contract, the formula is not to be reviewed until April 2006. The majority of the formula is to be applied to the four countries within the United Kingdom. The formula will be applied to practice populations, rather than PCO populations.

There is a suggestion from the medical press that Professor Carr-Hill has submitted manuscripts for publication to explain the workings and rationale behind the Carr-Hill formula.

Minimum Practice Income Guarantee (MPIG)

Initially, after the calculations were made using the Carr-Hill formula it emerged that 70% of practices would be worse off under this formula. As a result of further negotiation by the GPC of the BMA, a Minimum Practice Income Guarantee

(MPIG) was introduced to safeguard against this and that practice income did not drop off in the transition from the Red Book (1990 GP contract). The guarantee states that all practices will gain money under the proposed deal, providing doctors meet minimum quality levels.

The Global Sum is then compared to the Global Sum Equivalent (GSE), which is described in the next section, to decide if a correction factor is required and so implementation of the MPIG.

In order to try and understand how your Global Sum payment is comprised it is necessary to bear in mind the following figures.

1   The Global Sum (GS) – calculated using the Carr-Hill formula. As detailed above this is based on the practice population weighted for factors that influence needs and costs.
2   The Global Sum Equivalent (GSE) – this is based on a single year of previous fees paid under the 1990 contract Red Book. These fees have been uplifted to 2004/05 prices.
3   Correction factor (CF) – this is the difference between the GS and the GSE. If the GSE is greater than the GS, then this correction factor is added to the Global Sum allocation.

The Minimum Practice Income Guarantee is the sum of the Global Sum and the correction factor. Therefore: MPIG = GS + CF.

If the GS is greater than the GSE, then the MPIG factor does not apply. As a practising GP the most perplexing aspect of these formulas is trying to understand how they have been calculated and to ensure that the practice is no worse off financially as a result. The GSE is easier to calculate as a practice can refer to the last year of payments from their PCO. However, this is not so straightforward for the Carr-Hill formula and the GS.

> **Practical point**
> After 1 April 2004, it should only be the Global Sum that will change as a result of an altering list size and not the correction factor.

There have been reassurances made that the MPIG is a permanent guarantee to ensure equitable payments to practices in line with the previous 1990 GP contract and that the MPIG will be available as long as any practice requires it. In other words it should protect those practices that lose out as a result of the redistributive effect of the new resource allocation Carr-Hill formula.

Temporary residents

There is one further factor that affects this calculation. Once the final figure is arrived at, a figure for temporary residents is then deducted based on a one-year aggregate of fees paid to GMS practices for treating temporary residents. The figure is added to the Global Sum, but where the correction factor is positive this is then deducted from the Global Sum Equivalent.

Calculation of the Global Sum Equivalent (GSE) figure

The Global Sum Equivalent (GSE) figure is calculated according to the Statement of Financial Fees and Allowances (SFA) payable to GPs from the 1990 contract referred to as the 'Red Book'. The fees that comprise the GSE are as follows:

- capitation fees
- basic practice allowance (BPA)
- cervical cytology targets (half)
- child health surveillance
- new patient registration fees
- night visits
- out-of-hours allowance
- adult vaccinations and immunisations (excluding influenza)
- contraception
- maternity (excluding intrapartum care)
- emergency and immediately necessary treatment fees
- PGEA
- minor surgery (one-third)
- rural practice payments
- superannuation (employer's share)
- deprivation payments
- health promotion
- arrest of dental haemorrhage
- staff reimbursement budget including superannuation, training and locum nurse fees
- GPs' superannuation deductions.

Indicative Contractor Budget Spreadsheets (ICBS)

Based on this information PCOs should be able to provide Indicative Contractor Budget Spreadsheets, and so yet another new acronym, ICBS.

A particularly helpful website in finding out more about these calculations is the NHS Confederation website: www.nhsconfed.org/gmscontract.

The argument that has been given for the variations in Global Sums is that with any new formula there are winners and losers and that this income protection (MPIG) will be built into the new contract for at least two years. It is anticipated that this correction factor will continue for perpetuity and so for as long as it is needed and that it will only change if there is a formula review. MPIG should mean that all practices will start the new contract from a neutral or improved position in terms of this basic funding. It will fluctuate with changes in the population: for example, the list size of a practice. Furthermore, it is not the only source of income as the rest of this book will explain as there are payments for enhanced services and quality indicators.

Checking if your Global Sum figure is correct

As the Global Sum forms a core part of a practice's income, it is important to ensure that the practice is not losing out; the ICBS should be read carefully and the appropriate person in a PCO approached if a practice has any questions. For those practices receiving the MPIG and correction factor, to calculate the GSE, they should refer to the practice's previous income under the 1990 contract for the baseline period which is: 1 July 2002 to 30 June 2003 (uplifted to the 2004/05 value). It is important to state that the following do not comprise part of the GSE calculation:

- asthma and diabetes management
- chronic disease management
- childhood immunisation targets
- quality allowance or initiatives
- seniority payments
- intrapartum maternity care
- minor surgery (two-thirds of the payment)
- cervical cytology (half of the payment).

The GSE should include the employer's contribution to superannuation and the recent rise to 14%.

It was argued by some that this could be likened to 'sticking plaster' and that the MPIG removes the incentive to provide a wider range of services. Indeed, it has the potential to allow practices with many patients who provide limited services to earn more than those providing higher quality care. In the meantime the GPC is reviewing the funding formula and hopefully this will be completed before the formula becomes operational in April 2004.

Cash to Accruals Conversion

It is possible that the income of practices receiving the MPIG may be cut as a result of the 'Cash to Accruals Conversion' and this is the subject of a BMA notice of 26 May 2004. This adds further complexity to an already complex calculation. Accounts by PCOs are to be drawn up on an accruals basis and so deal with the amount of money due to contractors (GPs) in the year 2002/03 regardless of when it was received. However, as payments to individual GPs under the 1990 GP contract were outstanding or paid late the GSE equivalent calculations will be made on the money a practice actually received in the 2002/03 year (baseline period), rather than what they should have received. This means that GSEs will be multiplied by a factor of 0.9956, effectively cutting this figure by approximately 0.5%. This subject is still being discussed at a national level by the GPC of the BMA.

Other issues relating to the Global Sum

Where will all the money come from?

Where is the money going to come from to potentially pay GPs more? The allocated budget from primary care is to increase from £6.1bn per annum in 2002/03 to £8bn in 2005/06. This will facilitate the projected uplifts to the Global Sum, increases in quality payments and enhanced services. New resources to be delivered under the new contract will be protected through a Gross Investment Guarantee

(GIG). The GIG ensures that the new resources promised in 'Investing in General Practice' will be delivered.

Practical point
Current gross fees and allowances have been uplifted by 3.225%.

A BMA letter of 19 September 2003 provides details of the UK-wide quality preparation lump sum payment of approximately £9000 per average practice based on its patient list size.

In order to be paid the Global Sum a practice must provide core or essential services and additional services.

Core (essential) General Medical Services

- Management of acute illness, including health promotion advice and referral.
- Chronic disease management.
- Palliative/terminal care.

Additional services

These are normally expected of all practices; an opt-out is possible, but a sum of money will be subtracted from the Global Sum as a result. The PCO will look to commission these 'additional services' from another practice and thus an opt-back-in may not be possible by the practice if they later change their mind. Additional services comprise the following:

- child health surveillance
- contraception (excluding IUDs)
- obstetrics (antenatal and postnatal, but not intrapartum)
- childhood vaccinations (plus target payments)
- cervical screening
- basic minor surgery (cryotherapy and curettage).

Appraisal

This is a further fee that is under negotiation. Prior to 1 April 2004 there was a fee paid to the appraisee for the time taken for the appraisal process and locum cover to provide protected time for the appraisal itself. Similarly there should be a fee for the appraiser who conducts the appraisal, the time out of practice for the appraiser and the time taken to arrange the appraisal and to read the paperwork. In addition, there is still a question as to who will pay for the appraisal of salaried doctors and locums, previously referred to as 'non-principals'. Will these fees comprise part of the Global Sum? Tracing the source of these payments may be blurred as PGEA arrangements and the collection of 'PGEA points' has been replaced by appraisal and PDPs.

Over-75 and three-year 'checks'

When the new contract was negotiated there were to be no more compulsory annual over-75 or three-year health checks which came about as a result of the 1990 GP contract. There was to be 'no carry-over' from the Red Book or GP Terms of Service and the new contract was to reward workload and quality. Similarly, there would be no payments for health promotion or chronic disease management which were introduced in the 1990 GP contract and these would appear under the essential core services within the Global Sum and also some of the quality indicators of the Quality and Outcomes Framework.

Out of hours

Perhaps one of the biggest and most fundamental changes of the new contract is the choice to opt out of out-of-hours responsibility for the cover of patients registered with the practice which includes Saturday morning surgeries. The responsibility will pass to the PCO and each GP will have to pay approximately £6000 for this. The figure will be 6% of the Global Sum.

Claims for locums

In relation to reimbursement of locum costs, the GP concerned has to be away sick for at least one week. The locum concerned must not be a partner or an employee of the practice, unless it is a job-share situation, and prior agreement must be obtained from the PCO if reimbursement is to be claimed. All the necessary documentary evidence will need to be supplied such as a medical certificate and any accident compensation must be offset against the cost.

It is expected that PCOs will continue to provide locum payments for single-handed practices and those in job-share arrangements where a GP is sick or on leave as detailed below.

The actual amount for reimbursement remains relatively low and appears to be based on old capitation rules in the 'Red Book' which relate to the number of patients a doctor is expected to cope with before extra locum assistance is required. This is based on a workload of GPs from a long time ago and does not take into account their additional workloads involving health promotion and chronic disease management. The fee amounts to £948.33 per week which is a 6.5% rise on the 'Red Book' and is to cover the costs for partners on the following types of leave:

- maternity
- paternity
- adoption
- sickness
- long-term sickness.

For the parent who is not the main carer, adoption and paternity leave is for a two-week period. For the parent who is the main carer the figure of 26 weeks will be the same for adoption leave.

For GPs where prolonged study leave (PSL) is granted for up to 12 months, practices may be entitled to an educational allowance of £129.50 a week and a contribution up to £948.33 per week towards the cost of employing a locum. This figure will differ if the GP concerned on PSL is part-time (*see also* pp. 151–2).

Practical point
PCOs will retain the right to award practices less or refuse to meet their locum costs. In addition, a PCO is permitted to offer its own locum as an alternative to the practice employing a locum of their choice. This option cannot be refused without a good reason and PCOs have the right to withhold locum payments if this situation arises.

Previous arrangements for appraisal and locum cover for appraisal should be included under the Global Sum and may not be itemised separately.

CHAPTER 3

Enhanced services and Directed Enhanced Services

These are a series of optional 'extra', more specialised innovative services which GP practices – through GPs, nurses and other allied healthcare professionals – may choose to provide. Finance has been made available for these enhanced services through the new contract and also for some enhanced services to move some care that is currently in secondary care into primary care. Some of the care provided may fall into the province of GPs with Special Interests (GPswSIs). Enhanced services will be commissioned by the PCO, but there is no obligation for practices to provide these enhanced services.

Enhanced services fall into three categories:

- Directed Enhanced Services (DES)
- National Enhanced Services (NES)
- Local Enhanced Services (LES).

PCOs will be free and able to commission whatever enhanced services they consider appropriate to meet local health needs above a guaranteed minimum level of investment. In essence PCOs can be viewed as providers and may seek GP practices to provide those services. These services will be performance managed by the SHAs or equivalent corporate bodies and should reward innovation.

In relation to any enhanced service it is important for each practice to think about what they are currently doing and whether that equates with one of the defined Directed or National Enhanced Services as detailed in:

BMA Publication, *New GMS Contract 2000: Investing in General Practice. Supporting Documentation.*

Furthermore, the practice should consider whether it is going to be financially worthwhile to provide or continue to provide that service and also if the practice has the necessary staff and facilities to provide such an enhanced service.

The differences between Directed, National and Local Enhanced Services

What are the differences between Directed, National and Local Enhanced Services?

- DESs are essential services over and above those defined as part of the Global Sum, but provided to a higher national specified standard.

- NESs are additional services over and above those defined as part of the Global Sum, but provided to a higher national specified standard.
- LESs are local additional innovative services over and above those defined as part of the Global Sum, but provided to a higher specified standard that are to be piloted and evaluated.

They are all specialised services undertaken by GPs or nurses in primary care and services that are at the primary/secondary care interface and may enable the movement of some services from secondary into primary care. They are services that will address specific local health needs within the practice or the area served by the PCO. As well as these services providing a local requirement they will have considerable impact on the income of a practice.

The specifications for the DESs and NESs were published in May 2003 in the second contract document as detailed above.

Directed Enhanced Services

These services are obligatory for PCOs to provide and PCOs will be keen to commission individual GP practices or clusters of GP practices to provide these services.

These services are under national direction with national specifications and benchmark pricing which all PCOs must commission to cover the PCO's population. They are also some of the 'additional' services detailed in the Global Sum but are delivered to a higher standard, for example extended minor surgery. They include the following and are services that one might usually expect GP practices to provide:

- improved access
- quality information preparation
- childhood vaccinations and immunisations
- influenza immunisations
- extended minor surgery (more than curettage, cautery and cryotherapy)
- care of violent patients.

Improved access

The NHS Plan aspires that by 2004 all patients can see a primary care practitioner if they wish to within 24 hours and any GP within 48 hours, i.e., not necessarily the GP of a patient's choice. There are obviously some caveats such as 24 or 48 hours referring to working days, i.e., excluding Saturdays, Sundays, bank holidays and designated staff training through defined protected learning time initiatives. Also, circumstances can be considered where consultations may be reduced, e.g., through telephone consultations, but the target will be assessed against waiting time for a face-to-face contact. There are also variations for the access targets in the four different countries of the UK.

In the case of emergencies patients should be dealt with quickly or immediately in accordance with clinical need. However, it should be appreciated that the understanding by patients and healthcare professionals of the differences between 'emergency', 'urgent' and 'routine' may be different and this should be acknowledged.

Some smaller practices have always offered advanced access by running 'open surgeries' where patients can arrive and queue to see a GP without an appointment. However, the regulations state that as well as seeing a GP within 48 hours there should also be a 'booked' appointment.

There are arguments for and against this DES and a recent article in the *British Journal of General Practice* entitled 'Access – who needs it?' states:

> One result of this policy is that it tends to give priority to those patients whose clinical need is lowest. Another is that it tends to provide a poorer service to those whose need is greatest. (Fitzpatrick M (2004) *British Journal of General Practice.* **54:** 485.)

For those who wish to find out more about the possible advantages and disadvantages of this DES, a further paper appears in the same journal: Salisbury C (2004) Does Advanced Access work for patients and practices? *British Journal of General Practice.* **54:** 330–1.

Advanced access can halve waiting times (Pickin M, O'Cathain A, Sampson FC and Dixon S (2004) Evaluation of Advanced Access in the National Primary Care Collaborative. *British Journal of General Practice.* **54:** 334–40). Views as to its impact on overall workload differ between GPs.

A question that some practitioners may ask is whether government initiatives such as NHS Direct and walk-in centres will duplicate these services instead of, as Fitzpatrick suggests, targeting the hard-to-reach groups. A further potential problem with this new DES is that it has the potential to affect both choice and continuity of care by reducing the facility for advanced bookings and having a choice of GPs. And for many patients this is a priority rather than advanced access. It is important therefore that practices do not restrict patients to same-day or next-day appointments.

Practical point
Practices need to achieve a balance between reducing the backlog of appointments and supporting 'today's work today'.

It is important to monitor daily capacity and changes in demand. Points that practices should bear in mind are:

- identifying other methods of meeting demand
- implementing new practice.

A plan for implementation needs to be agreed with the local PCO for this DES. Practices should therefore consider collecting the following information as evidence of providing this enhanced service.

1 Detailing the current situation in a practice – this will require systematic recording of the number and nature of appointments requested.
2 Monthly data which demonstrates improvement. (Some PCOs may ask for information on the third available appointment as a measure of access to GPs and other healthcare professionals within the practice.)

3 Random audits of next available appointments to ensure continuous achievement of the targets and so maintenance of the system.
4 Contingency plans and the employment of locum staff if required for holidays
   and sickness.
5 Quarterly review to include a capacity and demand audit, the effectiveness of
   any contingency plans and to demonstrate any improvement.

More than 5000 practices are using the National Primary Care Development
Team's advanced access methodology to design appointment systems to help them
better manage demand and improve access (*see* www.npdt.org). Also nearly all
practices have reached the targets of seeing a primary care practitioner within 24
hours and any GP within 48 hours, which has a political imperative (The NHS
Plan for 2004) driving it. This DES has been commissioned to meet these targets in
2003/04 and is planned to run until 2005/06.

Practical point
For practices having difficulty implementing the system in their practice,
there should be a PCO access facilitator available to advise.

Remuneration for this DES will be £5000 per annum per average practice of 5891
patients and like all DESs there should be an annual uplift of 3.225%. In addition,
there are 50 bonus points under the Quality and Outcomes Framework (QOF) for
the maintenance of this national access target. This is not time-limited and is
discussed in Chapter 7. The date that this target has to be reached by for the QOF
is 31 December 2004. Practices should also have received a payment if they were
successful in achieving improved access targets for the period immediately prior to
the new contract and so meeting the NHS Plan targets.

Quality information preparation

A clear protocol needs to be agreed with the PCO outlining the way the practice
intends to summarise patient records on-site. A model protocol should be available
from each PCO. Inevitably this may necessitate a practice to employ a summariser
or summarisers which could be an additional expense to a practice.
   Summarising requires a sound plan or protocol that needs to be carried out to
completion. This needs to be discussed within the practice, then agreed with the
PCO and then concluded between the summarisers and the practice prior to
commencing the project.
   The following could comprise such a protocol.

a Organising and pruning records in preparation for summarising by a
   summariser.
b Read coding significant clinical events on the practice computer system.
c Archiving conditions that are of less significance.
d Deciding how sensitive information will be recorded.
e Organising how new information will be summarised and inputted (ongoing
   summarising).

f   Role of clinical staff, in particular GPs or a lead clinician, in the summarising process.
g   Training and supervision of the summarisers.
h   Ensuring confidentiality and signing of a confidentiality clause by summarisers.
i   Where the summarising process will take place and access to a computer terminal.
j   Monitoring the summarising process – lead clinician comparing a selection of notes to the computer summaries.
k   The role of scanning in the archiving process.
l   A timeframe for the initial process.

It should also be noted that there is some overlap with the QOF and four quality indicators (Records 14, 15, 18 and 19 under the organisational domain of the QOF – Records and Information about Patients). This DES prepares for these quality indicators as it is a time-limited enhanced service to be offered for two years and so is to be completed by 31 March 2005. The following quality indicators are relevant.

- Records 14 (3 points) – The records, hospital letters and investigation reports are filed in date order or available electronically in date order.
- Records 15 (25 points) – The practice has up-to-date clinical summaries in at least 60% of records.
- Records 18 (8 points) – The practice has up-to-date clinical summaries in at least 80% of patient records.
- Records 19 (7 points) – 80% of newly registered patients have had their notes summarised within eight weeks of receipt by the practice.

Practical point

This demonstrates the further worth of this activity in relation to the QOF as it will assist in the creation and maintenance of disease registers and so income generation.

Summarising can be done by doctors, practice nurses, other healthcare professionals, medical students, appropriate PCO personnel or by commercial companies employing any of these. Those who act as summarisers need to be trained so that they can recognise the importance of information from the patient records and then which associated Read codes are used to code that clinical information. Staff must be trained by those with summarising experience or by the GPs in the practice. It is important that summarisers have access to doctors in case of queries or the doctor designated to liaise with the summarisers.

Practical point

Practice managers should be aware that it is recommended that trained summarisers do not work more than six hours a day and that records should not be taken out of the practice and that summarisers have on-site access to medical records and the practice computer.

Practices who seek to be commissioned for this DES will be required to produce an annual review with the following information:

1   the number of completed summaries
2   average time taken to conduct a summary
3   how records are being maintained following summarisation
4   the expenses generated by the summarising process.

Summarising is not a new activity for many practices. GP training practices have had to achieve clinical summaries in 80% or more of their patients. However, this may not always have been computer summaries, but a summary sheet at the front of the written records. Similarly, this information has been required by fund-holding practices and latterly PMS practices in relation to budget applications. What information is important to summarise? The following are some likely important areas:

- significant illness/disease problems/disorders
- repeat/current medications
- matching repeat medications to medical conditions
- allergies
- vaccinations
- parameters such as smoking status and cessation advice, alcohol intake, height, weight, blood pressure, urinalysis, family history
- screening such as cervical cytology, mammography and PSAs (prostate, specific antigen).

In relation to the use of the practice computer for inputting information it may be helpful to see if the local PCO has a Primary Care Information Services (PRIMIS) facilitator. PRIMIS is a free service to PCOs to help them improve patient care through the effective use of their clinical computer systems. PRIMIS is funded by the NHS Information Authority and is based in the Division of Primary Care at the University of Nottingham (www.primis.nhs.uk).

The finance available for this process seems inadequate considering the task required. PCOs will offer an annual budget between £1000 and £5000 for the average practice with a population of approximately 5500. Assuming a practice had not summarised any records this could equate to an approximate reimbursement ranging from 20p to £1 if the process were completed in 12 months. There should also be money available to all practices for general quality preparation and through the attainment of the quality indicators referred to.

Some practices have already completed or started the notes summarising process. In 2003/04 to 2004/05, where funding is needed the benchmark price will be between £1000 and £5000 per average practice (population around 5500); practices with less or more patients will receive a percentage reduction/increase, depending on the need for the activity. This money is additional to funding that will be available to all practices for general quality preparation and the continuing provision for summarising and the maintenance of records through the QOF. It is not therefore intended to cover the full cost in those practices that have not yet undertaken any summarising of their notes. These figures will be uplifted by 3.225% in 2004/05 and 2005/06.

> **Practical point**
> Some practices may argue that these summaries can be handwritten on paper records. A recurrent theme in this book is the need to Read code all information on the GP practice computer system as all other aspects of the new contract and financial claims are dependent on this information. Similarly audits requested by the PCO to demonstrate that targets are being met will require the use of a computer and associated search facilities.

Payments and preparation for delivering quality

Every practice should have received a lump sum payment in 2003 to help them prepare for implementing the QOF of £9000 for the average-sized practice. This is the Quality Preparation Payment (QPP). There should be a further payment of £3250 in April 2004.

There should also be a Quality Information Preparation Payment (QuIPP) which applies to the Quality Information Preparation DES and is made via this DES. The payments should be between £1000 and £5000 for the two years 2004/05 and 2005/06 (*see* opposite).

Quality payments will be adjusted according to national average practice list sizes, known as the Contractor Population Index (CPI). The current CPI is as follows.

- In England divide the registered patient list by 5891 for GMS practices and 5907 for PMS practices. In Wales divide by 5885, in Scotland by 5100, and in Northern Ireland by 4914.

The suggested use by the Department of Health (DoH) for these payments is as follows:

- upgrading practice IT systems (e.g. with new GMS-compatible software and templates)
- summarising and ordering notes onto the computer (QuIPP)
- training staff and doctors on correct use of new Read codes for the QOF
- training on use of the computer generally
- payment of locums to allow staff to attend away days on the new contract
- funding external consultants to facilitate practice business planning around the new contract.

Childhood vaccinations and immunisations

Given the recent controversies, e.g., in relation to the MMR (measles, mumps, rubella) vaccination, this may be a difficult DES to deliver. Why? There is a requirement to maintain the targets of the last 1990 GP contract to undertake to immunise children under the age of five years with the relevant immunisations based on the existing lower (70%) and higher (90%) target payments.

In essence there is no change from the old contract and practices are finding these increasingly difficult targets to achieve and so to provide adequate immunity against preventable childhood diseases such as measles as a result of the recent MMR controversy.

For practices wishing to offer this DES, the following national guidance should be used as the basis for plans to submit to the PCO.

1   a practice register of all eligible children up to five years of age for the childhood immunisation and preschool booster programme
2   making parents/guardians of children on the register aware of the available immunisation programme
3   providing the relevant immunisations
4   providing trained staff to deliver the DES (and the use of local Patient Group Directives – PGDs)
5   provision of on-site resuscitation equipment
6   entry of immunisations in patients' records, refusals or adverse reactions
7   an annual review of the immunisation programme through audit.

Payments available for providing this DES are as follows.

● Childhood immunisation lower target: £2655.
● Childhood immunisation higher target: £7965.
● Preschool booster programme lower target: £822.
● Preschool booster programme higher target: £2465.

However, these prices are based on a practice with a list of 5000 patients, which has 59.25 patients aged two years and 61.45 patients aged five. The prices detailed above are multiplied by the ratio of actual patients in these age bands to the number of patients provided above. The prices will be uplifted by 3.225% per annum.

As under the previous 1990 contract practices will be able to claim target payments based on the percentage of children that fall into the defined age groups who have been immunised on the first day of each quarter.

Practical point
Exception reporting, including for informed dissent, does not apply for this DES.

Influenza immunisations

Although this is a DES, similar to the childhood immunisation and preschool booster programme, this is both an 'item of service' and target achievement scheme similar to the previous 1990 GP contract. However, unlike the previous contract there should be no disparity between PCOs as there is now a national agreement to reward this activity which annually and traditionally is undertaken by GP practices.

The purpose of this DES is to provide influenza immunisation for those aged 65 and over and other at-risk groups. This is to reduce the serious associated morbidity and mortality from influenza by immunising those most at risk and so avoid patients being hospitalised. So what's involved?

First, to keep a register of those at risk patients:

1   aged 65 and over

and those patients with the following conditions:

2   asthma
3   chronic respiratory disease
4   chronic heart disease
5   chronic renal disease
6   immunosuppression
7   diabetes

and patients living in:

8   long-stay residential or nursing care.

Throughout the UK, the target for immunising those aged 65 and over is 70%. No uptake target has been set for immunising those in the non-age-related at-risk groups, but uptake should be maximised where possible in these at-risk groups. Existing arrangements in each of the four countries will continue to apply in terms of obtaining supplies of flu vaccine.

Practical point
Once practices have identified at-risk patients and those over 65 years, call and reminder systems for these patients on their list should be put into place.

The only group with a target of immunising over 70% is patients aged 65 and over. Immunisations given between 1 August and 31 March in the relevant year will count towards an item of service payment that differs for England, Scotland, Wales and Northern Ireland in the at-risk groups. It is expected, but not obligatory, that most immunisations will be given between 1 September and 31 January.

The national DES specification details the following criteria to be met for practices aspiring to provide this service and submit plans under each of these items to their PCO:

i   the development and maintenance of a register
ii   a call and recall system
iii   use of standardised Read codes.

In relation to Read codes, practices are advised to Read code the following information on the practice computers in relation to the patients for whom an item of service payment is being claimed:

• invitation letter for immunisation
• administration date of the vaccine
• no consent to vaccination (where vaccine is declined)
• contraindication to vaccination.

Payment will continue at the current existing rates in each country, uplifted by 3.225% per annum until such time as a stock order system is in operation across the UK. In England the same rate will apply for under 65s at risk as for the over 65s. In Scotland, the rate for under 65s will be an item of service fee of £6.80, uplifted by 3.225% per annum. (Readers should check in *MedEconomics* and with their PCO for the up-to-date fee.) Income can also be generated for influenza vaccination quality indicator points under the QOF discussed in Chapter 6.

Practical point

The understanding of the author is that to gain the fee for those patients over 65 years of age who are not also in an 'at-risk' group, the 70% target will need to have been reached for the practice. Practices should check this interpretation with their PCO.

In Scotland the fee will be partly determined on creating a register of those under 65s at risk to allow consideration of an early move to a sliding scale, including those patients over the age of 65. GPs should check with their local Health Boards for further details.

Pneumococcal immunisation

When providing immunisation against influenza it is also worth providing a simultaneous immunisation against pneumococcal infections which are responsible for a high percentage of serious chest infections. (It is not recommended for children under two years unless the conjugate pneumococcal vaccine is given.)

Immunisation against the pneumococcus bacterium is recommended in the following groups:

- over-65-year olds
- post-splenectomy patients
- those with diabetes
- immunocompromised and HIV-infected patients (human immunodeficiency virus)
- people with chronic liver disease or alcoholism
- people with heart failure
- chronic renal disease or nephrotic syndrome patients
- chronic lung disease patients, e.g., with chronic obstructive pulmonary disease (COPD)
- patients with cochlear implants.

(This information is taken from www.gpnotebook.co.uk where further details may be found.)

Practical point

As influenza vaccination is a DES, PCOs can choose whether to keep the service within general practices or whether to award the service to outside providers. Pneumococcal vaccination is not part of this DES, but may attract an item of service fee from some PCOs.

Extended minor surgery

Cryotherapy, curettage and cauterisation will continue to be done under the additional service of minor surgery paid through the 'Global Sum'. However, there is an opportunity for GPs with skills in dermatology and associated surgical skills to undertake the following procedures and claim payment as a Minor Surgery DES:

1   injections of muscles, tendons and joints
2   invasive procedures, including incisions and excisions
3   injections of varicose veins and piles.

In order to conduct any of these procedures and claim payment for them they should be conducted by a practitioner within a practice who has 'the necessary skills and experience to carry out the contracted procedures in line with the principles of GPs with Special Interests (GPswSIs)'. Such practitioners would need to be able to demonstrate:

- competence
- a sustained level of activity
- regular audit of minor surgery
- appraisal on this specialist activity
- regular continuing education in the speciality.

In addition, practices undertaking minor surgery should fulfil the following:

- adequate facilities
- nursing assistance
- appropriate sterilisation and infection control procedures
- record of fully informed consent
- appropriate use of pathology services
- audit of clinical outcomes, rates of infection and follow up of malignancies
- ensuring that relevant information reaches the patient's records whether in the practice or where the procedure is being undertaken for another practice.

In relation to payment, a PCO will agree with the practice the basis on which this Minor Surgery DES will be funded and whether there will be an upper limit as there is with present minor surgery claims. It is anticipated that payments will be of the order of £40 for a joint injection and £80 for 'cutting surgery'. However, this is a particular DES where some PCOs are describing funding difficulties. These prices will be uplifted by 3.225% in 2004/05 and again in 2005/06.

Care of violent patients

The need for this DES has arisen for patients who have been removed from a practice list as a result of aggressive or violent behaviour. This is an important initiative of the new contract to protect GPs and their staff against violent patients by the provision of a designated service.

There is a need to provide a stable environment for continuing general medical services for these patients so that they can receive continuing healthcare. Once a practice makes the decision to remove a patient from their list as the result of violent, abusive or disruptive behaviour they should notify the PCO and if appropriate the police. The PCO should inform the chosen DES provider for violent patients and ensure that their records are transferred immediately.

A practice that decides to provide care to such patients under this DES would need to do so on a long-term basis (minimum of 12 months) to adequately address their health and social needs.

Practical point

The practice should be aware that they are taking on a potential risk and dangers.

Such a DES needs an appropriate incentive to ensure a safe environment for the practitioners involved in giving that care for people who are potentially and repeatedly violent. A PCO would need to explore with a practice the additional support that might be required to provide these facilities safely.

Such patients often have complex and wide-ranging health and social care needs and it can be difficult to provide the wider range of facilities that practices would usually aspire to. Review of their future care would need to be on an annual basis.

Care of violent or potentially violent patients is a specialist area of general practice and would involve liaison with the following groups:

- PCO
- LMC
- social services
- police
- transport to avoid home visits.

Safety is paramount and other services may need to be involved, e.g., for patients with personality disorders. The hope of providing a DES for violent patients is that the patient and doctor may work constructively together leading to an improved doctor–patient relationship.

Practical point

Practices wishing to provide a DES for violent patients should discuss this further with their PCO. Given its specialist nature and the facilities and resources required, it may be that a PCO chooses and commissions one practice in the area to provide such care.

Payment

It has been recommended that a retainer fee of £2000 be made available with consultation fees of £40–80 during working hours with an increased fee out of hours of £50–100.

Further information

A useful website with more details about Directed Enhanced Services with examples of implementation and service level agreements is the National Primary and Care Trust Development Programme website: www.natpact.nhs.uk/cms/156.php.

CHAPTER 4

National Enhanced Services

All practices are expected to provide essential services and those additional services that they are contracted to provide to all their patients through the Global Sum and those services commissioned through DESs. National Enhanced Services (NES) have national specifications which outline the more specialised services that can be provided by practices.

The NESs include the following possible services:

- intrapartum obstetric care
- near-patient testing – monitoring of anticoagulation
- near-patient testing – for patients being treated with penicillamine, sulphasalazine, gold injections, auranofin or methotrexate for rheumatoid arthritis or methotrexate for psoriasis
- IUCD and IUD insertions
- specialised sexual health services
- specialised alcohol misuse services
- specialised drug misuse services
- specialised depression services
- specialised services for patients with multiple sclerosis
- care of the homeless
- immediate care and first response
- minor injury care.

The specifications of these services are designed to cover the enhanced aspects of clinical care of the patient, all of which are beyond the scope of essential services as stated in the 'Blue Books'. No part of the specification by commission, omission or implication defines or redefines essential or additional services.

The differences between DESs and NESs

DESs are essential services over and above those defined as part of the Global Sum, but provided to a higher specified standard. NESs are additional services over and above those defined as part of the Global Sum, but provided to a higher specified standard. They are not therefore directed but, like the national specifications of DESs, there is set or 'benchmark' pricing.

Funding of NESs

Difficulties arise where a PCO argues that a NES is part of a practice's essential and additional work that they have been contracted to provide and that they are already covered by the Global Sum. It is optional whether a PCO chooses to commission and provide these services in primary care. This can lead to dispute between individual practices and the local PCO as the GPC of the BMA has already negotiated and agreed that the NESs listed at the start of this chapter be recognised and reimbursed appropriately by PCOs using the benchmark pricing.

A good example of an NES which is a more specialised service beyond the scope of essential and additional work is the NES for Minor Injuries.

Yes, a GP can see a patient who has just suffered a head injury or stitch a laceration under the national standards defined under this NES or they can advise the patient to attend the nearest accident and emergency department that provides this service. Some GPs will argue that their goodwill has been exploited for too long and that provision of a quality minor injuries service should be rewarded appropriately. Therefore, it is important that practices are aware of the NESs that have been negotiated by the GPC of the BMA as part of the new contract and make their views known to the PCO if they have been informed that funding is not available for a NES.

Provision of NESs and appraisal

In order to provide any of these NESs, GPs must have a satisfactory annual appraisal and revalidation where they can demonstrate both competence and ongoing training to enable them to contract and deliver for each NES. The appraisal criteria will include both the generalist and special interest aspects of the work.

Practical point
It is expected that the level of training required for a GP providing an enhanced service is identified in the GP's personal development plan (PDP) and, where additional training is required, local mechanisms are found to address this in conjunction with the PCO.

Further information on NESs

Details specific to each NES are now summarised and further information or clarification may be gained from the BMA Publication, *New GMS Contract 2003: Investing in General Practice. Supporting Documentation.* These summaries have been produced from this national document together with the national documents available on the Department of Health website: www.dh.gov.uk.

Intrapartum obstetric care

Obstetrics is an area of clinical practice where women have indicated a wish to have greater continuity and a choice of maternity care in hospital or at home. It is government policy to promote such choice and continuity of care and where possible for a GP with the necessary skills to attend during the delivery is an extension of a mother's choice.

Most GPs no longer provide intrapartum obstetric care and under the previous 1990 GMS contract an extra item of service fee could be claimed for provision of this care. However, GPs in some rural locations may provide intrapartum care as the nearest specialist unit may be too distant to their practice. Some GPs with a Special Interest (GPswSIs) in obstetrics continue to provide hospital intrapartum care in a few maternity units and continue to attend selected home births with midwifery support. Overall intrapartum care provides continuity of care from a GP-led team.

Like all NESs there is a national specification to provide an enhanced service which is a specialised service beyond the scope of an essential general medical service. Therefore, in order for a practice to undertake this NES the following would be required which is assisted through the funding of the service by a PCO:

- a register of mothers receiving intrapartum care
- support of each patient and the nominated midwife
- provision of clinical skills:
  - maternal and neonatal resuscitation
  - induction of labour for post-maturity
  - interpretation of cardiotocographs (CTGs)
  - augmentation of labour
  - appropriate instrumental delivery
  - stitching of an episiotomy or a perineal tear
- stating the place of care, e.g., hospital or home
- maintaining an obstetric record
- consent for appropriate involvement of the necessary team of carers
- carefully following locally agreed guidelines
- ensuring fully informed choices and so consent
- evidence of continuing professional development (CPD) in the area and associated resuscitation skills
- annual review of care through audit
- representation in local relevant committees for making guidelines
- working with the local midwives and maternity unit.

Those GPs who provide the service must demonstrate appropriate experience, such as holding the Diploma of the Royal College of Gynaecologists (DRCOG), and would be subject to annual appraisal and revalidation.

Payment

This is £200 per patient and a further £50 for a neonatal check performed within 24 hours of the birth. This is a considerable increase in payment when compared with the 1990 GMS contract where a fee of £53.48 would be payable to a GP on a local obstetric list.

Near-patient testing

Near-patient testing (NPT) is the administration of medication and monitoring of side-effects through the performance of tests outside of the traditional hospital and associated hospital laboratory setting by the patient's GP practice. A good example of this, which can also be conducted by patients in their own homes, is the measurement of blood glucoses. However, NPT can include tests done in the hospital laboratory but acted upon by GP practices in relation to dosing medications or other clinically indicated actions.

There are many advantages to NPT as follows:

- immediate availability of results, e.g., glucose, International Normalised Ratios (INRs) and urinalysis
- quick turnaround time of laboratory results and associated patient management
- patient satisfaction.

Similarly, tests such as a full blood count (FBC) can be performed by the laboratory, where there is a particular need for a fast turnaround time associated with frequent patient monitoring – for example, some of the therapies used to treat rheumatoid arthritis. Regular blood monitoring is vital due to potentially serious side-effects that the associated medications can cause for conditions such as rheumatoid arthritis.

It is anticipated that medication side-effects can be significantly reduced if the necessary monitoring through NPT can be carried out in a well-organised way close to the patient's home, e.g., at the local practice rather than the hospital, where a patient could have to wait for an outpatient appointment.

Near-patient testing – monitoring of anticoagulation

Anticoagulation is increasingly being used in medical practice, particularly with the anticoagulant drug warfarin. It is more commonly being used in patients with:

- atrial fibrillation to reduce the incidence of embolism and so cerebrovascular accidents
- deep vein thrombosis (DVT) and pulmonary embolism (PE).

The aim of anticoagulation is to increase the bleeding time but this has to be balanced against the risk of haemorrhage. Therefore drugs such as warfarin have to be regularly monitored and the dose adjusted according to the INR which can be measured at hospital laboratories or using calibrated instruments at GP practices.

GPs involved in deciding the dose of warfarin that patients are taking should be familiar with its indications and risks. Also they should be familiar with different INR ranges for different conditions and have a method in place to stop warfarin when the suggested duration of anticoagulation has been completed. However, for some patients treatment may be indefinite, e.g., those who have had a heart valve replacement.

To gain funding for an anticoagulation NES the following criteria should be fulfilled:

- maintaining a register for patients receiving anticoagulation
- call and recall, appropriate professional links and referral
- education of newly diagnosed patients
- individual management plans
- patient-held record, record keeping
- audit and an associated significant event log

- staff training
- hospital admissions or deaths must be reported to the PCO within 72 hours.

Payments are at four levels.

- Level 1 – Prescribing of warfarin by the practice as advised by secondary care where investigation, e.g., a blood test, its interpretation and dosing of medication is made by a secondary care specialist service (£6–10).
- Level 2 – Prescribing and dosing of medication following interpretation of investigation(s) by the practice where the blood test is taken outside of the practice (£75–100).
- Level 3 – Same as level 2, but using a practice-funded phlebotomist (£80–110).
- Level 4 – Same as level 3, but where the practice undertakes the laboratory test using appropriate equipment (£85–120).

An additional fee of £3.50 may be payable if a house visit is necessary to perform the service.

These figures are per patient per year for those patients who are on the register for being anticoagulated with warfarin.

Near-patient testing – in rheumatoid arthritis and psoriasis

This is for patients with rheumatoid arthritis being treated with any of the following medications:

- penicillamine
- sulphasalazine
- gold injections (sodium aurothiomalate)
- auranofin
- methotrexate

or patients with psoriasis being treated with:

- methotrexate.

Regular monitoring of these medications through NPT and so the appropriate blood tests is required to reduce the incidence of their potentially serious side-effects. Such NPT should result from initiation of therapy by a specialist in secondary care where the duration of therapy is defined and reviewed on a regular basis. The care should therefore be shared with secondary care. For this NES, a practice would be required to fulfil the following criteria:

- maintenance of a register with a suitable recall system and details of the indication for treatment, its duration and the date of the last appointment in secondary care
- education of newly diagnosed patients and their carer and provision of continuing information

- providing individual management plans
- appropriate shared care arrangements and referral as clinically indicated
- training of staff
- adequate record keeping
- annual review
- notification within 72 hours to the PCO clinical governance lead of an emergency admission or death that is or may be due to the medication that is being monitored
- accreditation of practitioners providing this NES who undergo annual appraisal and revalidation.

For each of these medications prescribed, there should be a protocol that details dosage and monitoring regimes. As a general rule all patients should have the following blood tests prior to treatment:

- full blood count (FBC)
- electrolytes and renal function (urea and electrolytes – U&Es)
- liver function tests (LFTs).

All patients require urinalysis prior to treatment except in the case of medication with sulphasalazine.

There are also specific additional monitoring requirements for each medication as follows.

- Penicillamine – FBC and urinalysis every two weeks for the first eight weeks of treatment and then at monthly intervals except where there has been any dosage increment when they should be undertaken after a week.
- Sulphasalazine – FBC and LFTs should be conducted at three, six and 12 weeks after the initiation of treatment and then at three monthly intervals. If a patient becomes unwell an urgent FBC should be taken and interpreted appropriately.
- Gold injections (sodium aurothiomalate) – FBC and urinalysis is required prior to each injection and an ESR (erythrocyte sedimentation rate)/CRP (C-reactive protein) can be helpful when judging possible response to treatment.
- Auranofin – FBC and urinalysis should be taken every fortnight for the first three months of treatment and then on a monthly basis.
- Methotrexate – FBC should be taken weekly for the first six weeks of treatment and then monthly. However, if the medication is increased there should be a FBC after a week. LFTs should be taken every three months and U&E and creatinine every six months.

Payments are at four levels:

- Level 1 – Prescribing of medication by the practice as advised by secondary care where investigation, e.g., a blood test, its interpretation and dosing of medication is made by a secondary care specialist service (£6–10).
- Level 2 – Prescribing and dosing of medication following interpretation of investigation(s) by the practice where the blood test is taken outside of the practice (£75–100).

- Level 3 – Same as level 2, but using a practice-funded phlebotomist (£80–110).
- Level 4 – Same as level 3, but where the practice undertakes the laboratory test (£85–120).

An additional fee of £3.50 may be payable if a house visit is required to perform the service.

These figures are per patient per year for those patients who are on the register for rheumatoid arthritis or psoriasis who are being treated with the drugs listed at the beginning of this section.

Intra-uterine device (IUD) fittings

Approximately 5% of contraceptive usage in the UK is through intra-uterine contraceptive devices (IUCDs). In other countries such as those in Scandinavia, the figure is as high as 20%. Clinical issues relating to the use of IUCDs are as follows:

- clinical effectiveness of IUCDs is excellent
- a failure rate exists for all devices of 0.2–2.0 per 100 woman-years
- association with relatively high levels of litigation related to failure and fitting
- the levonorgestrel-releasing intra-uterine system also decreases menstrual loss
- insertion of a copper IUCD up to five days after presumed ovulation can be used for emergency postcoital contraception.

IUCD fitting is not undertaken by all GPs and expertise in IUCD fitting needs to be maintained. Litigation is associated with differing levels of professional competence in relation to insertion as well as problems during insertion.

The aims of this NES are to provide:

i a full range of contraceptive options
ii levonorgestrel-releasing intra-uterine systems to treat menorrhagia
iii availability of emergency postcoital contraception using IUCDs.

This NES will fund:

i fitting, monitoring, checking and removal of IUCDs as appropriate
ii production of an up-to-date register of patients fitted with an IUCD and the device fitted (this is to be used for audit purposes, and to enable the primary care team to target these patients for healthcare checks)
iii regular CPD
iv provision of adequate equipment for IUCD fitting
  - an appropriate room fitted with a couch and adequate space
  - equipment for resuscitation
  - a variety of vaginal specula and cervical dilators
  - equipment for cervical anaesthesia
  - the presence of an appropriately trained nurse for the patient and the doctor
v chlamydia screening should be undertaken prior to IUCD insertion. If positive, referral for screening of other sexually transmitted infections (STIs)
vi the use of condoms to prevent infection

vii a check of the IUCD after fitting (it is suggested that this takes place at six weeks and thereafter annually; any problems such as abnormal bleeding or pain should be assessed urgently)

viii provision of written information at the time of counselling and after fitting of the IUCD in relation to follow-up and the symptoms about which patients should seek urgent medical attention

ix adequate recording of the patient's clinical history
   – the counselling process
   – results of any chlamydia screening
   – the pelvic examination
   – problems with insertion
   – type and batch number of the IUCD
   – follow-up arrangements

(where a patient is not registered with the practice, the practice providing this NES should ensure that the patient's registered practice is given all appropriate clinical information)

x the use of a levonorgestrel-releasing intrauterine system for the management of menorrhagia as part of an agreed local care pathway

xi Annual review with:
   a patient register
   b continuous usage rates
   c reasons for removal
   d complications.

Negotiations are taking place to ascertain if contraceptive implant insertion can be funded as part of this NES, e.g., for etonogestrel subdermal implants.

Accreditation

Practitioners undertaking this procedure should have undertaken appropriate training. This should be based on modern, authoritative medical opinion, for example the current requirements set down by the Faculty of Family Planning and Reproductive Healthcare (FFPRHC) for the letter of competence in intra-uterine techniques (LoC IUT). This involves:

• a demonstration of gynaecological skills in assessing the pelvic organs
• a minimum number of ten observed insertions in conscious patients
• appropriate knowledge of issues relevant to IUCD use, including counselling.

Other doctors who can be considered as professionally qualified to provide this NES include doctors:

• who have previously provided IUCD services
• who satisfy at appraisal and revalidation that they have the necessary continuing medical experience, training and competence.

Payments

In 2003/04 each practice contracted to provide this service will receive a £75 insertion fee per patient and a £20 annual review fee per patient. These prices will be uplifted by 3.225% annually for 2004/05 and 2005/06.

Specialised sexual health services

There has been a substantial increase in high-risk sexual behaviours in the UK over the last ten years which some sources have referred to as a 'sexual health crisis'. This is for the following reasons.

- Since 1995 STIs including HIV have risen.
- Diagnoses of chlamydia, gonorrhoea and syphilis have doubled in the last five years.
- Teenage pregnancy rates in the UK are the highest in Western Europe.

Sexual 'ill' health is therefore a significant health concern. Although sexual health services have been defined as an NES, it could be argued whether or not it should be an 'essential' service under the new contract. Furthermore, open access contraceptive services through family planning clinics and sexual health services through genito-urinary medicine (GUM) services are overstretched and there will be much sexual health need that is currently unmet. Taking the example of chlamydia, which is the most common bacterial STI in the UK, this can cause pelvic inflammatory disease, infertility and ectopic pregnancies. As a result, it is anticipated that there will be a national Chlamydia screening programme in place by 2008.

The following are good reasons why primary care should deliver sexual health as an NES:

i   primary care provides about 75–80% of contraception
ii one-third of chlamydia infections are diagnosed in primary care
iii access to primary care is excellent
iv training can be targetted in primary care.

Service outline

The delivery of this NES should be informed by relevant national strategies and also those providing the service locally to each PCO and the needs of that population. It is particularly important to take into consideration the following:

- prescribing issues
- drugs of limited value
- attendance
- follow-up rates
- hepatitis B testing
- immunisation rates
- partner notification.

Plans for local sexual healthcare should involve liaison with all providers and relevant agencies and these should be part of the audit process of this NES.

This NES will fund:

i   HIV testing, including pre- and post-test counselling
ii   STI screening
iii the practice as a resource to colleagues in sexual healthcare
iv appropriate training and CPD
v   liaison with local sexual health services including cytology and microbiology laboratories
vi record keeping on the advice, counselling and treatment provided
vii a register of all patients being treated under the NES
viii appropriate arrangements for review
ix costs of condoms, pregnancy testing kits and other additional resources
x   treatment of STIs without prescription charge
xi effective communication with all young people including young men, gay and lesbian people, and ethnic minorities
xii a holistic approach to assessment of risk of STI, HIV and/or unplanned pregnancy, including consideration of other relevant health problems
xiii provision of information on, testing and treatment for all STIs (excluding testing and treatment of HIV infection, syphilis, hepatitis B and C or treatment-resistant infections)
xiv partner notification of relevant infections
xv a sound understanding of the role of different professional groups in the shared care of HIV-positive patients, and those at risk of HIV
xvi suitable training for all staff involved with patients seen for sexual health and HIV-related conditions
xvii all practices undertaking this service will be subject to an annual review which could include an audit of:
    a the number of patients seen for specific interventions
    b the number of people screened and treated effectively
    c attendance rates for each service offered
    d gestation at termination of pregnancy and follow-up contraception rates
    e the number of at-risk individuals tested and immunised according to local guidance for blood-borne viruses
    f age, gender, sexuality and ethnicity of patients to ensure that those most at risk from unplanned pregnancy and poor sexual health are accessing the practice offering the NES.

Accreditation

Those doctors who have previously provided services similar to the proposed enhanced service and who satisfy at appraisal and revalidation that they have such continuing medical experience, training and competence as is necessary to enable them to contract for this NES can be considered as appropriately qualified to do so.

Payments

In 2003/04 each practice contracted to provide this service will receive an annual retainer of £2000 plus an annual payment of £200 per HIV-positive patient (paid quarterly in arrears) and £100 per other patient (paid quarterly in arrears.) These prices will be uplifted by 3.225% annually for 2004/05 and 2005/06.

Specialised alcohol misuse services

This NES outlines the more specialised services to be provided for those patients who suffer with alcohol dependency, which may affect 4% of the population or more.

GP practices have the opportunity to intervene early with these patients given adequate facilities. This is particularly important as it is believed that patients who could be referred to as 'problem drinkers' consult their GPs twice as often as other patients. Furthermore, it has been estimated that 0.7 million men and 0.6 million women drink at 'risky' or 'hazardous' levels. Consultations relating to alcohol problems are recurrent and it is painful to witness the destruction of patients' lives with alcohol problems, some of whom are relatively young. It is not an easy condition to treat despite the involvement of specialist services. The relapse rate is high and those with dependency delay seeking help, and it is a problem that should be screened for in primary care.

Why is it important to intervene early with this group of patients? Alcohol misuse is associated with a range of physical and psychiatric health problems. Also it is believed that up to 65% of all suicide attempts are linked with excessive drinking. In addition, alcohol is a major contributor to accidental death. Alcohol-related illness is an area that requires a proactive approach, not least during secondary school years and to professional groups. Alcoholism is not a new problem. An issue of the *New Zealand Medical Journal* of 1903 describes 'the treatment of inebriates in special institutions'.

Screening for those with alcohol problems in general practice is a possible way of reducing subsequent illness. However, practitioners should be aware of a meta-analysis that suggests that only two or three patients per thousand screened will benefit from the hard work entailed in screening. (Beich A, Thorsen T and Rollnick S (2003) Screening in brief intervention trials targeting excessive drinkers in general practice: systematic review and meta-analysis. *BMJ.* **327:** 536–42.)

Indicators that might lead one to suspect that a patient has an alcohol problem could be:

- feeling the need to reduce alcohol intake
- irritation when drinking is criticised
- guilt about one's consumption
- the need to drink in the morning
- regularly smelling of alcohol during working hours
- exhaustion and symptoms of depression
- repeated mistakes and complaints, disciplinary action or loss of job
- recurrent irritability and temper outbursts
- poor relationship with colleagues
- domestic disharmony.

The aim of this NES is to improve the quality of treatment of these patients by ensuring practices have the funding and adequate staff and training and where treatment is beyond the scope of essential services.

In secondary care, one in seven acute hospital admissions are thought to be alcohol related. Brief interventions can reduce alcohol consumption by over 20% and so reduce the number of patients who become dependent on alcohol. Alcohol is also a significant contributory cause of:

- hypertension
- stroke
- heart disease
- oral and upper gastrointestinal cancers.

This NES will fund:

i   a register of all patients who admit they are alcohol misusers
ii   practices to undertake brief interventions and offer support to carry out behavioural change
iii   follow-up treatment including counselling sessions or referral to local alcohol services or attendance at a day programme or residential rehabilitation centre
iv   detoxification regimes
v   routine use of assessment tools
vi   liaison with local specialist alcohol treatment services
vii   appropriate training
viii annual review which could include an audit of:
    a   those identified and recorded as alcohol misuse patients
    b   the advice and/or treatment offered to patients who, following screening, have been shown to misuse alcohol
    c   the number of patients who have reduced their alcohol consumption
    d   feedback from patients who misuse alcohol and their families.

The funding for this NES emphasises that those with alcohol problems need to be taken seriously and, as well as involving the GP, specialist help is likely to be required. Local alcohol teams have a vital role as relapse is common. Self-help groups, e.g., AA (Alcoholics Anonymous), play an important role.

Accreditation

Doctors who may be considered as appropriately qualified to run this NES are those who have previously provided similar services to that outlined. In addition, they must appreciate that it is a condition where therapeutic outcomes may have limited success as a result of relapses, but success may be through such an NES bearing in mind that GPs are often the first point of contact in this common condition. Also they can satisfy at appraisal and revalidation that they have the necessary continuing medical experience, training and competence to provide this enhanced service.

Payment

In 2003/04 each practice contracted to provide this service will receive an annual retainer of £1000 plus an annual payment per patient (paid quarterly in arrears) of £200. These prices will be uplifted by 3.225% annually for 2004/05 and 2005/06.

References

Charlton R (2003) Tips on colleagues with alcohol problems. *BMJ.* **326:** s114.
Charlton R (2003) Read, reflect, respond section. *Learning Resource 16 – Tips on colleagues with alcohol problems.* 5 November (www.bmjlearning.com).

Specialised drug misuse services

Drug misuse and its complications are a considerable problem nationally and internationally. An estimate has been made that the number of drug users in the UK is in the region of 150 000–200 000. However, it is difficult to be precise, but most practices will have patients registered who are drug misusers. There is a higher prevalence in inner cities and urban areas in comparison to rural areas.

In relation to health, there is wide-ranging harm and ill-health associated with drug misuse, some of which can be fatal. This includes blood-borne viruses such as different types of hepatitis and HIV. Regarding blood-borne viruses the major route of transmission in the UK is by sharing injecting equipment such as blood-contaminated needles and syringes. In addition to physical dependence and associated problems, there are also mental health problems, of which a small proportion of individuals commit violent crimes.

This NES refers specifically to drug misuse, but it may also be helpful to define the term 'substance misuse'. Substance misuse is defined as the misuse of alcohol and/or other substances including illegal drugs, solvents and over-the-counter medicines.

Practical point

There is therefore a considerable overlap between the terms of drug misuse and substance misuse and an NES is likely to incorporate the more general term of substance misuse.

A 'dual diagnosis' can be defined as the occurrence of a drug or substance misuse problem and mental illness in the same patient at the same time. There are conflicting views on how many people in the UK may be suffering from such a dual diagnosis and are in need of treatment. Estimates have been made that more than half of those using mental health services have a dual diagnosis and are frequently young men. Further information may be found on the following website: www.drugscope.org.uk.

A person with substance misuse problems is much more likely to have an additional mental health problem and vice versa. In considering this NES specifically in relation to drug misuse, there is likely to be co-existing ill-health relating to physical, emotional, psychological and/or social problems and there may also be associated accommodation and legal problems. For practices undertaking this NES, these health needs need to be addressed as far as possible.

> **Practical point**
> For several of the NESs it is worth remembering the World Health Organization (WHO) definition of health:
>
> > Health is a state of complete physical, mental and social well-being and not merely the absence of disease or infirmity.

In order to be considered to provide this NES, a practice would need to have the following in place:

i   an accurate register of patients who misuse drugs
ii   an appropriate review process
iii   safe and secure practices
iv   ability to demonstrate effective liaison with local drug services and other relevant agencies and knowledge of local detoxification procedures
v   links with:
      – local pharmacies
      – primary care drug support workers
      – social services
      – the Child Protection Service
      – local mental and clinical health teams.

This NES will fund practices to:

i   develop and co-ordinate the care of drug users and develop practice guidelines
ii   treat dependent drug users with support from:
      – shared care drug service
      – GPswSIs
      – nurses with specialist interest
      – specialist providers
      (treatment will include the prescribing of substitute (opiate and non-opiate) drugs or antagonists using best practice as outlined in the DoH's drug misuse clinical guidelines or equivalent)
iii   ensure that prescribing takes place with a holistic approach taking into consideration other physical, emotional, social, psychological and legal problems
iv   audit prescribing practice
v   act as a resource to practice colleagues
vi   provide additional training and CPD
vii   maintain the safety and training of clinical and non-clinical staff
viii provide care for patients outside their own registered list (if this is agreed).

The NES will be subject to the following audits on a six-monthly basis:

i   audit of prescribing of substitute medication if appropriate and adherence to the local minimum standards
ii   audit of hepatitis B screening and immunisation data relevant to this patient population.

Annual review should include the following:

i   attendance rates
ii non-attendance rates
iii review against outcomes
iv financial review.

Accreditation

A practitioner providing this NES in drug misuse should have the skills to:

i   identify and treat the common complications of drug misuse
ii   carry out an assessment of a patient's drug use
iii provide harm reduction advice to a current drug user or his or her family
iv   test (or refer for testing) for other viruses, including HIV, and immunisation for hepatitis B to at-risk individuals
v   provide drug information to carers and users as to the effects, harms and treatment options for various common drugs of use
vi   assess, and refer appropriately, patients for drug misuse substitution treatment
vii utilise the range of commonly used treatment options
viii be aware of local policy
ix   work in an appropriate multidisciplinary manner.

Doctors who wish to be accredited and run this NES will require the above skills and will need to have previously provided similar services. They will also need to satisfy at appraisal and revalidation that they have the necessary continuing medical experience, training and competence. They will need to demonstrate that they are familiar and up to date with local and national guidelines.

Payment

In 2003/04 each practice contracted to provide these services will receive a £1000 annual retainer, £500 withdrawal treatment per patient per annum, and £350 maintenance treatment per patient per annum, paid quarterly in arrears. These prices will be uplifted by 3.225% annually for 2004/05 and 2005/06.

Specialised depression services

It could be debated whether or not this is a specialised service or one that GPs provide as part of their essential general medical services. It is also a common illness managed in primary care with only severe cases being referred to specialist services. It can also be a difficult condition to diagnose and one that patients would prefer not to acknowledge or be 'labelled' with.

It is reported that about 10% of people attending a GP practice have depression and up to one-third of the population will at some time have a milder form of depression. It can affect people at any age from childhood onwards and is more common in women, particularly during the postnatal period, older patients and in areas of social deprivation. Furthermore up to 5% of adults have a major depressive illness at any one time.

The aim of this NES in care of depression is to allow GPs more time to devote to patients with suspected or diagnosed depression. Also to provide further training to care for those with depression and in its recognition. For a patient to be entered into this NES, their depression should be diagnosed using a combination of evidence-based diagnostic tools, e.g., validated screening questionnaires, as well as specialist clinical judgements.

Symptoms of depression might include:

1 low mood most of the day
2 anhedonia – the inability to gain pleasure from normally pleasurable experiences
3 decreased appetite and weight loss
4 insomnia or hypersomnia (excessive sleepiness)
5 early morning wakening and difficulty getting back to sleep
6 shortness of temper, or irritability
7 fatigue on waking or reduced energy which improves as the day goes on
8 feelings of worthlessness or inappropriate guilt (which may be delusional)
9 diminished ability to think or concentrate or indecisiveness
10 tearfulness, becoming emotional or upset for no particular reason
11 anxiety and intrusive upsetting thoughts
12 recurrent suicidal ideation.

Why might such an NES be needed? There may not be a community mental health team locally or one that has a short waiting list. This NES would then be able to fill the gap in care so that patients with depression are treated as quickly as possible to gain the necessary and specialised service required for depression.

Funding for an NES in care of patients with depression is intended to cover the following:

- a disease register
- ensuring a multidisciplinary approach
- use of non-drug treatments such as Cognitive Behavioural Therapy (CBT)
- use of validated screening questionnaires
- adequate training for members of the primary healthcare team (PHCT)
- individual health plans
- referrals as appropriate
- annual review to include audit with a particular emphasis on the medication used
- patient feedback using standardised questionnaires.

Payment

Practices providing this NES will receive an annual retainer of £1000 and an annual payment per patient (in arrears) of £80–100. These prices will be uplifted by 3.225% annually for 2004/05 and 2005/06.

Specialised services for patients with multiple sclerosis (MS)

The majority of people with MS stay in remission. However, around 15% of people have a form of MS that is known as chronic progressive MS with steadily worsening symptoms and progressive disability. It is perhaps true to say though that the natural history of the condition is never the same in two people and symptoms may differ as do the parts of the body affected. Symptoms vary in severity and duration, mild and short-lived or severe and long lasting. For some patients with MS their symptoms may lie somewhere in between.

Symptoms can include:

- double vision or blurred vision
- ringing in the ears or hearing problems
- numbness in the hands, arms, feet or legs
- giddiness and loss of balance, especially in the dark
- memory problems with poor concentration
- anxiety and depression
- fatigue especially in hot weather
- weakness, difficulty in walking and muscle pains and spasms
- speech difficulties
- problems with bladder and bowel control
- sexual problems.

There are 1 in 1000 individuals with MS and 3–7 per 100 000 new cases occurring each year. It is 50% more common in women than men.

Different members of the PHCT that can help:

- the GP
- district nurses
- counsellors
- physiotherapists
- occupational therapists
- continence advisers
- dieticians
- social workers.

MS is a condition with profound physical, psychological, emotional and social impact and a key role of the PHCT is to help people affected with the associated emotional and practical difficulties and their families and carers. Specialist care may also be required and care is likely to be shared with secondary care. Respite care may also be required on occasions for those severely affected.

To achieve this NES, it is expected that the practice and associated PHCT will work closely with the patient and their carers and any support services. Proactive healthcare should be provided to patients with MS.

This NES for more specialised care of patients with MS focuses on patients' health needs by working closely with the patient's carers. This NES has recognised the need to proactively address health problems for those who suffer with MS.

Provision of this NES requires:

- maintenance of a register
- a nominated lead co-ordinator
- regular assessment and medication review
- continued training in MS
- carer support
- individual health plans for each patient
- liaison with social services and secondary care
- an annual multidisciplinary review.

GPs who provide these services to MS patients will need to satisfy annual appraisal and revalidation.

Payment

For each patient with MS that receives this NES there will be a payment of £90–140 per annum which will be paid quarterly in arrears. These prices will be uplifted by 3.225% annually for 2004/05 and 2005/06.

Care of the homeless

Surveys suggest that the number of people who are homeless is increasing. Defining homelessness can be difficult and many individuals may fit this category where they have no secure home and are entitled to help from the local authority. People who are homeless may be individuals who:

- sleep rough
- stay in hostels or night shelters
- are bed-and-breakfast residents
- are squatters
- stay temporarily with friends or relatives.

A lack of consensus on the definition of homelessness has made it difficult in estimating the true figures of the number of people who are homeless, as well as the characteristics of homeless people as detailed above. One figure quoted on the 'Off the streets and into work website' in 2001/02 was 118 360. In London the total number was 31 130. There has been a year-on-year increase since 1997/98. A small proportion of these are those who sleep rough (www.osw.org.uk). The 'Crisis' website (www.crisis.co.uk), the national charity for solitary homeless people, suggests that there are around 380 000 single homeless people in the UK. About 504 people in England sleep outside on any one night, 267 of whom are in Greater London. These figures have been provided to give the reader a scale of the problem as it is difficult to obtain precise data.

Health problems in this group of people differ, but it is known that they are at greater risk of both physical and psychological illness, infectious disease e.g. tuberculosis, alcohol and drug abuse. Their health needs can therefore be complex and require a dedicated approach by practices with a specialist interest.

As providing for the health and social needs of this group of people is a specialised area, GP practices wishing to provide this NES will need the necessary training and knowledge. If they already have experience of working in this field this may help provide for this NES and should be discussed with the local PCO commissioning this NES. In addition, the GP practices will need to work closely with the relevant housing and social services.

By making this an NES four issues are addressed:

1 homeless people have equity of access to healthcare
2 it is possible to provide this group of people with continuity of care who have complex health needs
3 practices will be designated as having the knowledge and skills in this area
4 practices will work with relevant associated services and agencies.

Commissioning of an NES for the care of the homeless by a PCO is intended to fund practices to:

- keep a register
- liaise with local services including hospital accident and emergencies (A&E) departments
- participate in local homelessness forums
- proactively promote health services to the homeless
- be flexible in relation to registration and appointments
- have good working arrangements with local pharmacies
- organise appropriate staff training and updates
- provide regular screening assessments
- provide outreach services
- use relevant guidelines on prescriptions
- refer appropriately to counselling and community psychiatric nurse (CPN) services
- ensure health promotion and harm minimisation
- facilitate specialist assessment as appropriate
- provide an annual review of the service including feedback, audit, the length and number of consultations and referrals.

Payments

Practices commissioned to provide this service will receive an annual retainer of £1000 and an annual payment per patient (paid quarterly in arrears) of £100. These prices will be uplifted by 3.225% annually for 2004/05 and 2005/06.

Immediate care and first response

In most areas of the UK, this is a service primarily provided by the ambulance services and paramedics. The service provides pre-hospital immediate care and first responder roles to victims of trauma, e.g., following a road traffic accident (RTA), and life-threatening illnesses, e.g., heart attacks. However, in some locations and certain clinical circumstances, an ambulance service or a paramedic may request the attendance and assistance of an appropriately trained GP at the scene of a clinical emergency. This would be to give clinical support and skills beyond those normally expected and practised by GPs or paramedics.

The use of volunteer doctors at the scene of emergencies is nothing new. Some of these schemes started in the 1970s when ambulance staff had only very basic training. With significant changes to their training there has been a change in the role of both the ambulance service and that of the immediate care doctor. They work together, complementing each other's skills and abilities, to provide an extremely high standard of care.

Currently where GPs provide an immediate care/first responder role, their assistance is through a variety of structures, either as an individual commitment, a practice commitment or through commitment to an organised immediate care scheme. In some parts of the UK (although GPs currently receive no remuneration for the immediate care/first responder role), PCOs have fully funded the training of GPs for such work and ambulance services have been issued with relevant equipment and supplies.

This NES will fund providers to:

i   augment the ambulance service paramedics at the request of the ambulance service in the management of cases (actual or expected) such as:
   a   extended on-scene time or prolonged transit time to definitive care
   b   entrapment
   c   clinical or operational considerations exceeding the paramedic protocol, training or experience
ii   provide a trained response to immediate life-threatening illnesses within the accepted response times
iii provide rapid, skilled medical triage for multiple casualties
iv   provide trained Medical Incident Officers (MIOs) at the scene of major incidents
v   occasionally support the ambulance service during periods of extreme demand in meeting clinically critical target times
vi   log on or off call with control according to their other workloads
vii maintain and keep a copy of clinical records in accordance with the local format of the ambulance service.

Accreditation

Those doctors who have previously provided similar services to the proposed NES may seek to be commissioned by their local PCO. They would need to provide evidence at appraisal and revalidation of continuing medical experience in this field, together with appropriate training and competence.

Practitioners will normally be expected to:

i   as a minimum possess the Pre-Hospital Emergency Care Certificate (PHEC) of the Royal College of Surgeons of Edinburgh or other equivalent
ii   undertake a local orientation and familiarisation programme
iii undergo advanced driving tuition as required by the ambulance service
iv   undertake local communications systems training
v   undertake such refresher training as appropriate
vi   accept and obey the local statutory emergency service command structures

vii if the NES is operated locally through a local immediate care scheme, accept its rules and operational standards

viii maintain appropriate communications with the tasking control room concerning personal availability for call-out

ix be familiar with the scope and limitations of paramedic practice

x be willing to work in a team

xi accept the ambulance service tasking policy.

Practices or individuals who are contracted to provide such services should study the detail carefully regarding refresher training, CPD and the keeping of an individual log of incidents attended – in addition, the regulations relating to driving training and the vehicle that they use. This information is detailed fully in the BMA Publication, *New GMS Contract 2003: Investing in General Practice. Supporting Documentation.*

Payments

In 2003/04 GPs contracted to provide this service will receive an annual retainer of £1200 to £1500, the exact level depending upon whether equipment and supplies are provided by the PCO or funded by the practice, plus £60 to £90 per in-hours call and £120 to £150 per out-of-hours call. These prices will be uplifted by 3.225% annually for 2004/05 and 2005/06.

Minor injury service

The commissioning of a Minor Injuries Service (MIS) as an NES has the potential to take pressure off local hospital A&E services. Similarly, if PCOs do not recognise this as an NES that should be funded, then there is a potential for the reverse situation to apply.

Minor injuries or wounds usually refer to problems that are less than 48 hours old and may include the following:

- lacerations
- bruises
- minor dislocations of phalanges
- foreign bodies, including non-penetrative ones of the eye
- eye injuries
- injuries not amenable to domestic first aid
- head injuries without loss of consciousness
- burns or scalds less than one inch in diameter and excluding hands, feet, face, neck and genital areas
- minor trauma to hands, limbs or feet.

An MIS should fulfil the following criteria:

- initial triage
- assessment and immediate wound dressing if appropriate
- appropriate referral and follow-up
- adequate facilities including resuscitation

- provision of registered nurses
- infection control standards
- adequate patient information and consent
- use of histology services as appropriate
- maintenance of records and regular audit with appropriate peer review.

The following injuries are not appropriate for an MIS:

- where a patient cannot be discharged home after treatment
- penetrating injuries, e.g. of eye or abdomen
- artery, tendon or nerve damage
- history of loss of consciousness or collapse
- cardiopulmonary distress
- medication overdoses
- where a 999 call has been made for treatment.

GPs in a practice providing an MIS would be expected to have the necessary experience and training to satisfy relevant appraisal and revalidation procedures.

Payment

Providing such a service requires recognition of the cost. A practice that is contracted to provide an MIS should receive an annual retainer of £1000 and £50 for each minor injury that is managed. The PCO may place an upper limit on the number of claims that can be made, but this can be reviewed. In addition, all drugs, dressings and appliances should be funded and supplied by the PCO.

This NES has been a source of debate and not least over whether PCOs recognise this as an essential service or an NES. Depending on how individual practices interpret this under the new GP contract there is a potential for workloads to rise at local hospital A&E departments. Rural practices are put in a particularly difficult situation if PCOs will not fund this recognised NES as there may not be a hospital A&E department in near proximity.

CHAPTER 5

Local Enhanced Services

For the first time, the new GP contract enables PCOs to commission local services to meet local needs. Previously, the national 1990 GP contract allowed little flexibility in what services were provided locally, and to what specification. New, locally agreed contracts should ensure that patients, particularly those with long-term chronic diseases, have access to specialised services or treatments catering for a specific local need in primary care. These Local Enhanced Services (LESs) are commissioned by local negotiation, using the same structure and principles as NESs as detailed in the previous chapter to meet specific local needs.

Potential new LESs

It is anticipated that the GPC of the BMA will be drafting guidance for GPs who wish to bid for LESs based around the following service areas:

- asylum seekers
- non-English speaking patients
- patients with learning disabilities.

Other areas likely to be commissioned under the LESs could include:

- neonatal examinations within 24 hours of birth
- nursing home patient care
- area-wide in-hours home visiting schemes.

GPs with a Special Interest (GPswSI)

PCOs and GP practices will not be limited to this list and much may depend on needs in the locality and expertise of local practitioners. Some doctors may enter general practice with training in specialist areas in addition to vocational training in general practice. This will enable them to become a GP with a Special Interest (GPwSI) and they may be able to run a clinic for a local cluster of practices, therefore reducing the number of referrals and so cost of referrals to secondary care. This may also relieve the burden on secondary care of a high workload in particular specialities. Examples could be clinical areas such as:

- endoscopy
- urology
- dermatology.

Similarly, GPs could train to become GPswSIs and offer LESs to PCOs for possible commissioning. (The Department of Health in conjunction with the RCGP have produced guidelines for the appointment of GPswSIs to several areas of clinical care.)

The Quality and Outcomes Framework tends to cover important chronic diseases associated with high morbidity and mortality. However, it could be argued that many important conditions have been missed out of the framework and these will vary between localities and could form the basis potentially for LESs.

An important concern that doctors may experience is finding the necessary funding for such a service even though they can demonstrate a clinical need for the service. Even when funding is available and both small and large practices have bid for an LES where the clinical need has been identified and agreed with the PCO, it is still possible for a PCO to franchise out a service. This could be to a GP practice or it could be to an independent provider from the private sector where their bid has been more financially competitive or seen to provide a more comprehensive specialised service.

Clusters

PCOs are keen for practices to work together in clusters. There may also be an option for clusters to be involved in commissioning services. It may be financially beneficial for practices to work together on the principle of franchising services particularly in relation to the development of LESs. This could also include the setting up of specialist services by one or more PCOs, e.g., for postoperative care or leg ulcer care. This is also sometimes referred to as 'outsourcing' and could be something that is increasingly seen in the future as a result of the new contract. However, this could lead to further fragmentation of primary care services with patients being cared for by more than one primary care provider.

Development of an LES

As an LES would be based on the same principles as the DESs and NESs, a practice bidding for such an LES should adopt the existing NES specifications referred to in the last chapter as a possible template. It would be necessary to provide the clinical evidence and data to determine the design, size and scope of the service to be provided – also, to highlight the service protocols to facilitate the development of the service. If an LES is approved by a PCO it should be piloted and the necessary equipment funded.

Finance of an LES

If a PCO agrees to the provision of an LES, payment levels for LESs will also be agreed locally and not necessarily on a national scale as for DESs and NESs. Where an individual practice or cluster of practices believes there is a need and the expertise exists for a particular LES, it would be necessary to negotiate with the PCO for possible funding. If difficulties are experienced then practices should involve the LMC in the negotiations.

Practical point
Before setting up an LES, talk to the appropriate commissioning individual in your PCO about approval and financing the initiative.

Furthermore, it may be necessary to provide additional funding to help GPs prepare for appraisal and revalidation in relation to an LES and this could be an 'appraisal premium' that can be added to a practice's Global Sum. This premium should cover any training required by the appraisee and preparation time to set up the LES.

A further reason that PCOs may fund LES proposals are if they help them meet targets, e.g., for reducing referrals to secondary care.

Non-core services

It is apparent that some GPs are unhappy about continuing to provide services that they do not see as 'core' services, but have been having to provide 'free' under the previous 1990 GP contract. There are several of these non-core services that could meet the potential to be LESs as follows:

- depot injections of neuroleptics
- goserelin insertions
- etonogestrel implants
- phlebotomy services for secondary care
- arranging ambulances for hospital appointments
- postoperative care for early hospital discharges sometimes referred to as 'hospital at home' care including suture removal
- leg ulcer and wound care by practice nurses
- care of nursing and residential home patients.

A further non-core service in the future may be the proposals for the time-consuming electronic booking of hospital outpatient appointments when the necessary IT equipment and software is made available.

These are a few common areas that some practices regularly raise and there are also likely to be others. If practices are concerned about these issues they should speak to the relevant commissioning manager at their local PCO to see if a way forward can be found where this 'extra' work is rewarded through the financing of an LES or franchised out.

Practical point

LESs will be an important area of development under the new contract and practices need to maintain close communications with neighbouring practices in their cluster and the LMC to maximise the potential for developing appropriate LESs.

CHAPTER 6

Quality and Outcomes Framework: background, the clinical domain and exception reporting

When many people think of the new contract they think of the Quality and Outcomes Framework (QOF) as the major source of income. This is not the case. It is in fact the Global Sum. However, the QOF certainly has the potential to generate a considerable amount of additional income, but I have left it to the end of this book as it is not the only source of income and it is easy to overlook the other possible sources. The QOF is, however, the part of the new contract which forms a large proportion of the promised pay rise for GPs or 'new'/'additional' income and so reward for their 'extra' work. However, some doctors may argue that these targets are unrealistic and in some situations may not be achievable. Unlike the targets of the old contract, e.g., in relation to cervical cytology, it is possible to achieve a percentage of a target and so part payment through the attainment of quality indicator 'points'.

The QOF and the associated quality standards have been developed from many sources and negotiated by the GPC of the BMA. Sources include the NHS Confederation, the quality improvement models such as the Quality Team Development programme of the RCGP and the RCGP Practice Accreditation Scheme and the PRImary Care Clinical Effectiveness (PRICCE) scheme. The latter was piloted in East Kent using practice incentives starting in April 1998 to implement many of the organisational standards developed by the RCGP.

Role of the GPC of the BMA

On the BMA website the following statement appears:

> *The GPC aims to represent all GPs, to promote general practice and to protect its fundamental characteristics and interests.*

Focus on quality

Everything that is in the QOF requires to have an evidence base and not just that someone felt that it might be a 'good idea'. Quality indicators are specific and measurable elements of practice that can be used to assess the quality of care and have been derived from a well-researched evidence base. They may also therefore form some of the requirements of National Service Frameworks (NSFs). To demonstrate quality each indicator has to have an outcome and to look at outcomes each indicator must be able to be measured.

The good news for GPs is that, yes, the QOF is paid for and that providing these quality indicators through the QOF leads to reward in 'points' and so income to the practice. The big difference about the new contract is that the focus is very much on quality, rather than quantity, and so there are allowances made for not just the number of patients seen but the percentage of defined targets that are achieved. So the greater a practice strives for quality, the greater the reward.

Purpose of the QOF

It has been stated that the vision of the QOF is to raise the clinical and organisational standards in primary care based on best evidence. Some may debate whether this voluntary form of clinical governance contains the most important indicators and standards. For example, they may not always match existing targets set in the NSFs and by the National Institute for Clinical Excellence (NICE). However, this is not a question that this chapter will debate as these are the standards that have been chosen. The intention of the quality standards that are defined by indicators is that they should:

- reduce morbidity
- reduce mortality
- improve the patient experience.

Collecting points

Most readers will be aware that there are a total of 1050 points based on defined quality indicators that can be aspired to. The achievement of all of these points through the necessary conduct of clinical care and collection and input of data into individual practice computer systems is daunting to say the least. Yes, this might be achieved by paperless means, but the bureaucracy involved is almost exponential. To gain the income available a practice needs good organisation and management and co-operation from all the members of the team – in addition, a satisfactory PCO annual review to confirm that the claims made can be backed up by the necessary computer data.

The four domains of the framework

The whole document is called a quality framework which has been organised into four domains:

1   Clinical (comprised of ten chronic disease areas)
2   Organisational (five areas)
3   Additional services (four areas that can be chosen)
4   Linked payments (two areas relating to patient experience).

Quality indicators

Each area is subdivided into individual quality indicators where standards have been set which are the criteria that PCOs will audit for performance and so achievement of standards and how subsequent payments will be calculated. It should be stated that the indicators have varying levels of achievability starting with achievement levels as low as 25%. So a proportion of points may be attained as well as the maximum for a threshold of achievement of 90% as defined for some of the indicators.

Payments

By the time this book goes into print, GPs will have aspired to a proportion of the available 1050 points and then the difficult task is achieving this aspiration and hopefully more. Once this aspiration is agreed with the PCO, a GP practice will receive one-twelfth of the aspiration payment every month, which is one-third of the points aspired to. The remaining two-thirds pro rata or more will be paid after 12 months if it can be demonstrated that the aspiration (and possibly beyond) has been fulfilled or part fulfilled.

Points have a financial value. In the first year of the contract, the value of each point is expected to be £75.

Practical point

Although each point equates with £75, as practices are paid rather than individual GPs, the value of a point and so the proportion of this £75 varies with list size. In order to gain the whole £75, this equates with an 'average' list size of 5891 patients. If a practice has a list size less than this, the proportionate figure is paid per point achieved.

Similarly, as will be discussed later in this chapter, the number of points gained for an indicator varies according to the threshold that is achieved. For example, a minimum threshold may be 25% and the maximum threshold may be 90% to gain the full possible allocation of points for a clinical indicator.

Good news and payments

The good news is that although practices are being paid £75 per point from April 2004 it is anticipated that **this figure will rise to £120 per point from April 2005**. The QOF not only raises standards of good clinical practice, but also the income of a practice. Unlike the previous 1990 GP contract it is worth emphasising that practices will not miss out on the whole chunks of income simply by being half a per cent short of a required target. On the contrary the harder a practice works towards the QOF, then the greater the reward proportionally as they work towards the maximum thresholds.

Computer templates and Read codes

What is the key to success? Ultimately, not just the clinical work carried out, but its recording on the practice patient record computer system. Getting doctors to record information in a structured way during busy overbooked surgeries using computer templates is not easy. Each practice will need to devise a method to do this efficiently. For example, this may be the running of chronic disease clinics with appropriately trained practice nurses.

At the QOF PCO annual review, PCOs will audit patient data on the computer and in this way decide what payments are due. Theoretically, a scenario could arise where work has been done for the QOF, but has not been recorded on the computer and so a practice does not gain the income it has potentially earned. Furthermore, the templates used will need to employ the correct computer codes, referred to as Read codes. Previous computer templates used by a practice may not employ the correct Read codes and this can be checked with the software provider as to whether the necessary updates are available.

Practical point
PCOs will audit an individual practice's QOF outcomes and so points through entry of the correct Read codes. Practices who do not check that they are inputting patient data under the correct Read codes will lose income even though they have done the necessary work.

Read codes

Liverpool Health Authority provides a very helpful definition of Read codes. Read codes are a hierarchical classification system of clinical and administrative terms used on most GP computer systems as a means of recording information. They were created by a Loughborough GP, Dr J Read, and form the coding scheme favoured in the NHS which is in widespread use. The NHS Executive appointed Dr Read as the first Director of the Centre for Coding and Classification.

However, there appears to be little knowledge about what Read codes are and their structure – software supplier training does not normally cover coding. Many GPs are discouraged by the complexity of Read codes. Using the codes allows practices to:

- record data more consistently
- retrieve data with greater ease
- analyse/audit data
- communicate data to agencies, e.g., PCOs, using a common clinical language.

Discussing Read codes is important as data must be properly recorded and in GP practices this has many implications. Transfer of data relating to Read codes will be partly automatic using existing links to computer systems and also using an online interface with a national database called the Quality and Outcomes Framework Management and Analysis System (QMAS). PCOs will receive monthly data in this way that will help them with financial planning, e.g., in relation to the performance of practices in the QOF.

Make sure a template is set up for each of the ten chronic disease conditions in the clinical domain and that the template includes all the indicators that are correctly Read coded. A practice may also include any additional ones that the practice feels are important to the quality of care that they wish to provide. However, practices should be aware that this will not increase payments under the QOF.

It is possible to list all the Read codes for each individual quality indicator, e.g., for DM 2 – the percentage of patients with their body mass index (BMI) recorded – the Read code is 22K. Similarly for exception reporting, e.g., DM 15 where ACE1 (angiotensin-converting enzyme) inhibitors are contraindicated in the treatment of patients with diabetes or who have microalbuminuria or proteinuria and have had an adverse reaction to this medication. This Read code is 8128. However, the listing of all the Read codes would take up considerable space.

The Read codes for the QOF are available to view at the BMA website (www.bma.org.uk) or the Department of Health website (www.dh.gov.uk) or BMA Publication: *New GMS Contract 2003: Investing in General Practice. Supporting Documentation.*

Practical point

A decision that needs to be made by a practice is which individuals – for example, doctors or nurses, or the practice manager, or another designated individual – will input data into the computer – also, which individuals will keep a regular check on how the practice is performing in each of the four domains on a monthly basis.

Ignoring the framework

What if a practice chooses to ignore the framework, saying it is too busy as it is? Unfortunately, there is a penalty and the QOF is not entirely voluntary. Any practice failing to achieve at least 100 points in the first year of the contract and 150 points in the second year will have the equivalent amount of money deducted from their Global Sum. This is a further incentive to get to grips with the framework.

PMS practices will also be able to take advantage of the framework and this is discussed in Chapter 8.

We are informed that the government has invested £1.6 billion with an additional £1.9 billion into primary care. Why? There is evidence to suggest that there are aspects of primary care not being carried out to an optimal level, despite new guidelines and continuing medical education programmes. The QOF is therefore an incentive to do this, but finance is required to both run and reward this activity.

Practical point

For many years in primary care there has been a feeling by some people that practitioners have been counting things that do not matter. The new contract not only now rewards this 'counting activity' financially, but it is an opportunity to calibrate the quality of care that an individual practice is providing and thus counting things that do matter. For these two reasons it would seem unusual for a practitioner to wish to 'opt out' or ignore the QOF.

Clinical domains of the framework

There are ten clinical areas of the first domain of the QOF which relate to chronic disease management. These are listed in the following table, together with the number of available points. There are 550 clinical quality indicator points for the first domain.

Clinical Domain	Available points
Coronary Heart Disease	121
Stroke and Transient Ischaemic Attacks	31
Hypertension	105
Diabetes Mellitus	99
Chronic Obstructive Pulmonary Disease	45
Epilepsy	16
Hypothyroidism	8
Cancer	12
Mental Health	41
Asthma	72
Total	**550**

There are 1050 points in total and, so that readers can see at a glance what the other 500 points comprise, these are listed below.

Organisational Domain	Available points
Records and Information	85
Information for Patients (Communication)	8
Education and Training	29
Practice Management	20
Medicines Management	42
Total	**184**

Additional Services Domain	
Cervical Screening	22
Child Health Surveillance	6
Maternity Services	6
Contraceptive Services	2
Total	**36**

Patient Experience and Linked Payments Domain	
Consultation Length	30
Patient Survey	70
Holistic Care	100
Quality Practice	30
Access Bonus	50
Total	**280**

Total points (with clinical domain of 550)	1050

Potential income from the QOF

With £75 per point a practice with a defined average list size of 5891 could generate £78 750 for a total of 1050 points achieved. The actual figure paid by a PCO depends on the number of points achieved with a payment made proportional to the practice list size. For example, a practice with a list size of 2400 patients would receive a payment for 1050 points achieved of:

$$\frac{2400}{5891} \times 1050 \times £75 = £32\,082.84$$

If this practice aspires to gain all 1050 points and this is agreed with the PCO then an initial aspiration payment of one-third will be made = £10 694.28. This will be paid monthly for the year starting on 1 April 2004 at the rate of £891.19.

Disease prevalence and payment

Much of the QOF is complicated when it comes to payments and trying to calculate how much a practice is likely to be paid. This section is perhaps the most complicated in the book and yet vital to the understanding of how a practice gets paid under the QOF. And so, prevalence is a further factor to complicate this chapter.

The factor of prevalence has been introduced as prevalence of the ten chronic diseases of the clinical domain of the QOF varies from practice to practice and the Adjusted Disease Prevalence Factor (ADPF) requires to be calculated for each practice.

$$\text{The ADPF} = \text{the square root } (\sqrt{}) \text{ of } \frac{\text{Practice Prevalence}}{\text{National Prevalence}}$$

Let's take the example of a practice of 3000 patients which has 60 people with diabetes on the diabetes register and that 68 out of the potential 99 quality indicator points for diabetes have been achieved. Let's also assume that the National Prevalence for diabetes is 3%. The Practice Prevalence is 60/3000 = 0.02 or 2% and so below the expected National Prevalence.

The ADPF is the square root of 2/3 = 0.816

The payment the practice will receive is:

68 points $\times$ £75 $\times$ 0.816 $\times$ 3000 (practice list size) / 5891 (average practice size) = 68 $\times$ 75 $\times$ 0.816 $\times$ 3000 / 5891 = £2119.30

The theory behind this complex formula is that it is there to compensate practices with a low prevalence of a chronic disease to ensure that they are not under-resourced, and yet it does not adequately compensate those with a high prevalence. For example

- for a practice with a prevalence half the national average, the ADPF will be the square root of 0.5 which is 0.71

- for a practice where the prevalence is equal to the national average, the ADPF will be the square root of 1.0 which is 1.0
- for a practice where the prevalence is 50% above the national average, the ADPF will be the square root of 1.5 which is 1.2.

Furthermore, practices in the bottom 5% of the national range will have an uplift to the 5% level.

This formula has been the basis of considerable controversy as the payment received depends on both the Practice Prevalence and the list size. For example, a small practice with a high prevalence of diabetes, but the same number of people with diabetes as a larger practice and the same number of quality indicator points achieved, may receive a lower payment. It has been suggested therefore that a direct prevalence factor should be used rather than a square root. One assumes the same number of patients with diabetes in each of the two practices means the same workload.

It could be argued that a National Prevalence figure does not take into account variations locally and nationally in England, Wales, Scotland and Northern Ireland.

Practical point

Practices should be aware that Valentine's Day (14 February 2005) is the day that Practice Prevalence figures for the ten chronic diseases are calculated. These figures are used as the basis for prevalence calculations by the PCO in the financial year. This data will be collected through the Quality Management and Analysis System (QMAS) which will be a part of clinical IT systems of practices.

Audit: structure, process and outcome

The quality targets include all three principles of clinical audit – structure, process and outcome – and so it is important that these are identified for the QOF.

Structure means having an accurate patient disease register, e.g., for epilepsy, that is properly Read coded. When the PCO looks at the claims being made, local and national comparisons will be made with individual practices in relation to the percentage of each of the ten disease conditions to ensure that practices have included the expected number of patients on their registers. This means achieving the 'records' indicator.

Where an entry of a patient has been made 'recorded' in a disease register each entry should be looked at critically following a computer search. This is to find out which patients are on the register and to ascertain if there is evidence in the notes to support the diagnosis for all patients that are on the register or whether the disease register needs to be 'cleansed' accordingly.

Process means completing clinical management tasks and these could form part of the annual check or review as has been traditional with conditions such as diabetes.

Outcome means demonstrating quality against good defined standards of clinical care which may be difficult to achieve, e.g., a glycosylated haemoglobin (HbA1c) of less than 7.4% for patients with diabetes. One of the key aspects of achieving high quality scores is teamwork.

Practical point

Many patients will have their care shared between primary and secondary care and the two will need to work even closer together agreeing protocols of care. There needs to be a rapid, clear and accurate communication between the two about the delivery of such care and transmission of the outcome data of such care, e.g., blood test results.

Delegation and teamwork

The theory behind the new contract is that it should not further overload the already busy workload of the GPs in a practice. The emphasis is on each practice to deliver, which not only requires teamwork and delegating the work to appropriately trained nurses, but perhaps employing more individuals to undertake the extra work that is identified to meet the new quality standards set as 'targets' (thresholds).

Practical point

For each of the ten chronic disease conditions of the clinical domain, one person in a practice should take a lead role in setting up the process and oversee its effectiveness through repeated audit and monitoring.

The rest of this chapter discusses the clinical domain of the QOF and exception reporting and Chapter 7 discusses the other three domains and so the remaining 500 quality indicator points.

Clinical Domain

The clinical domain contains ten chronic diseases together with their individual quality indicators listed numerically. In this chapter, and Chapter 7, each chronic disease is abbreviated, e.g., CHD for Coronary Heart Disease and then the number of the quality indicator follows the abbreviation. Then a one to two word summary appears to alert readers to what the quality indicator refers to. Next to each quality indicator listed during the remainder of this chapter appears a sentence in italics that details the criteria that require to be recorded to gain points, e.g., smoking status. This sentence has been edited for this chapter and Chapter 7 and the exact text may be read in what is referred to as one of the two 'Blue Books' by BMA Publications: *New GMS Contract 2003: Investing in General Practice. Supporting Documentation.*

The author then interprets these criteria in a practical way for GPs trying to fulfil the criteria for the QOF. The 'Blue Book' above is helpful in placing the indicators into different categories, e.g., records (creating a disease register), diagnosis and initial management, and ongoing management.

Furthermore, for some quality indicators, e.g., asthma review, it may not be entirely clear as to exactly what is required by a practice to fulfil these criteria. **It is therefore important that this chapter and Chapter 7 are read in conjunction with this 'Blue Book'.** (This chapter and Chapter 7 are not an absolute reference to the new contract.) In the 'Blue Book', after the quality indicators for each chronic disease have been listed, three sections appear.

- The **'Rationale'** as to why each indicator has been selected for the QOF, e.g., national guidelines. The rationale also lists what might constitute a review, e.g., for Diabetes (DM) indicator 10 – neuropathy testing, it is recommended that sensation is tested using a monofilament or by vibration. This chapter could list all of these, but this would be duplication and take up many pages!
- **Preferred** coding – the Read code recommended for data entry on the GP practice computer system. For this indicator, which is neurological screening, the Read code is 68A1.
- **Reporting and Verification** – this defines the audit information that practices will be required to submit annually. Provided the information has been correctly Read coded and the disease register has been compiled, this task should be straightforward using the computer. In the example used, practices should be able to provide a report of the number of patients with diabetes who have had neuropathy testing in the previous 15 months. Verification refers to an identifiable source in the clinical record.

> **Practical point**
> The amount of clinical information that is to be recorded for the annual review may be at the discretion of local PCOs and should be checked with them so that future claims for points are not queried.

Coronary Heart Disease (CHD)

Of the ten clinical chronic diseases of the clinical domain this one has the most quality indicator points (121) and so emphasises the importance attributed to this common disease condition. In addition, there are points for other chronic diseases that are closely related including hypertension and diabetes. CHD is a multifactorial disease that includes general factors such as lifestyle, the environment and genetic predisposition. Specific risk factors include smoking, dyslipidaemias, obesity, hypertension, diabetes and a strong family history. Why is this clinical domain so important? This is because CHD is a major cause of both morbidity and mortality in the UK.

> **Practical point**
> Most of the ten chronic diseases in the clinical domain of the QOF are divided into the same sections, which include medical records and the creation of a disease register, diagnosis and initial management (which focus on smoking status and smoking cessation advice) and then ongoing management. This is an important point to bear in mind when creating or using computer templates.

There are 15 separate quality indicators: 12 with the abbreviation CHD for Coronary Heart Disease and three with the abbreviation LVD for the subset Left Ventricular Dysfunction (heart failure) with a total of 121 points.

Records

CHD 1. Disease register. *The practice is able to produce a register of patients with CHD (6 points).*

Many practices may already have such a register as work prior to the new contract has been underway in relation to aspirin therapy for this group of patients and the use of statins. However, there will be patients who are not on the register and should be. For those practices using a computer system, it is important to search for additional patients to go on the register who have a history of a myocardial infarction or angina and for patients taking medications that are commonly used to treat CHD. Their notes can be read to ascertain if entry to the register is appropriate.

Practical point

Creating a *disease register* for the first time means exploring several avenues to ensure that all patients with a chronic disease, such as CHD, are included on the disease register. It is expected that PCOs will compare the expected prevalence for a locality of an individual chronic disease with the reported prevalence of an individual practice. If it transpires that there is a considerable discrepancy between the two figures, then this could potentially affect the final payment given for quality indicator points claimed for that chronic disease.

Disease registers are basically part of the computer templates that relate to individual chronic diseases. This should vary on a daily basis depending on the practice developing a method to add patients with the disease who ought to be on the register but the information has not been inputted onto the practice computer or patients who are newly diagnosed. Each day correspondence and results relevant to patients with individual chronic diseases should be added to the relevant template. A computer search at defined intervals will access the register and where appropriate clinical data is absent a patient can be recalled for appropriate review. A lot is talked about exclusion criteria and so exemption, but it is important to sort out the inclusion criteria and which patients should appear on the disease registers in the first place. Exclusion criteria are discussed at the end of this chapter.

Diagnosis and initial management

CHD 2. Newly diagnosed angina. *The percentage of patients with newly diagnosed angina (diagnosed after 1 April 2003) who are referred for exercise tolerance testing (ETT) and/or specialist assessment (7 points). (Minimum threshold = 25%, Maximum threshold = 90%.)*

It is anticipated that many of these patients will have already seen a specialist or will have been sent to a rapid access chest pain clinic and so have had ETT.

However, for those patients who are entered on the register after 1 April 2003, it is important to document whether this has happened or not. (ETT can be used to detect ischaemic heart disease, to identify patients with reversible myocardial ischaemia who might benefit from revascularisation and assess prognosis of patients with CHD.)

Practical point
Minimum and Maximum thresholds are the targets necessary to achieve points. So how are they translated into income? The following hypothetical example may help. For CHD 2 above let us say that the threshold reached by a practice is 50% by the end of March 2005. The Minimum threshold percentage (25%) is subtracted from the percentage achieved (50%) which gives a figure of 25%. This is divided by the subtraction of the Minimum threshold percentage (25%) from the Maximum threshold (90%) and multiplied by the points available (7).

$$\frac{\text{Percentage achieved (50\%)} - \text{Minimum threshold percentage (25\%)}}{\text{Maximum threshold (90\%)} - \text{Minimum threshold percentage (25\%)}}$$

$\times$ points available (7) = 2.7 points

Therefore, 2.7 points has been achieved from the possible 7 points available.

CHD 3. Smoking status. *The percentage of patients with CHD, whose notes record smoking status in the past 15 months, except those who have never smoked where smoking status need be recorded only once (7 points). (Minimum threshold = 25%, Maximum threshold = 90%.)*

It is very important that this information is asked and recorded in the records of all patients at the practice as it provides an important basis for health promotion advice if the patient is a smoker and also this information is required for six of the chronic diseases of the clinical domain of the QOF. In addition, patients who have declared that they do smoke should perhaps be asked at consultations in the future whether they still smoke and whether they might like any advice in trying to stop.

Practical point
In relation to the new contract and good medical practice, there are certain pieces of information that most GP computer systems will alert the consulting doctor to, whether this information is required or needs to be updated on a summary screen. In relation to several quality indicators, smoking status is one of these and it is important that this information is collected when the opportunity arises as it may be that a particular patient is not seen again for 12 months.

CHD 4. Smoking cessation advice. *The percentage of patients with CHD who smoke, whose notes contain a record that smoking cessation advice has been offered within the last 15 months (4 points). (Minimum threshold = 25%, Maximum threshold = 90%.)*

Health promotion through advice to patients to stop smoking features recurrently in the QOF as it is a considerable factor in the aetiology of several diseases, not least CHD. Many practices have organised for their practice nurses to attend training courses to promote smoking cessation and so provide a structured treatment programme for patients who continue to smoke and are having difficulty stopping, but would like to stop. Investment in these training programmes and the allocation of nurse time to smoking cessation sessions will help practices meet many of their quality clinical indicators and improve the health of patients.

CHD 5. Blood pressure. *The percentage of patients with CHD whose notes have a record of blood pressure measurement in the previous 15 months (7 points). (Minimum threshold = 25%, Maximum threshold = 90%.)*

This is another indicator that features in four of the chronic diseases of the clinical domain of the QOF. In relation to health promotion and the prevention of heart attacks and strokes it is important to measure patients' blood pressures regularly and take appropriate action when repeated readings are consistently raised.

CHD 6. Blood pressure of 150/90 or less. *The percentage of patients with CHD, in whom the last blood pressure reading (measured in the last 15 months) is 150/90 or less (19 points). (Minimum threshold = 25%, Maximum threshold = 70%.)*

This is a difficult target to achieve and hypertension is frequently a factor and co-existing problem in CHD and it is important that it is controlled in order to reduce further morbidity and mortality. There will inevitably be some patients in whom it is difficult to gain adequate control and they are likely to fall into the 30% of people in the practice with CHD whose reading is greater than the required 150/90 for this quality indicator.

CHD 7. Cholesterol. *The percentage of patients with CHD whose notes have a record of total cholesterol in the previous 15 months (7 points). (Minimum threshold = 25%, Maximum threshold = 90%.)*

It has been known for some time that raised cholesterol levels are associated as a risk factor for the development and progression of CHD. It is important therefore that the disease register for CHD is used to recall those patients who have not had a cholesterol reading in the last 12 months.

Practical point

In order to meet the requirements of the CHD quality indicators it is important for practices to conduct an annual review of patients on this register and for other chronic diseases through a recall system where this is indicated. Although many of the quality indicators suggest 15 months, it is better to aim for 12 months, as it may take three months for a patient to attend the practice following recall.

CHD 8. Cholesterol of 5 or less. *The percentage of patients with CHD whose last measured total cholesterol (measured in the last 15 months) is 5 mmol/l or less (16 points). (Minimum threshold = 25%, Maximum threshold = 60%.)*

Once cholesterols have been measured on this patient group it is important to advise and provide the necessary treatment for those patients who have a total cholesterol greater than 5 mmol/l. Once treatment measures have been put in place, e.g., by prescribing a statin, it is desirable that the cholesterol level is rechecked to ascertain whether it has had the desired effect and if the person is compliant to taking the medication. Also the blood tests should be used to monitor liver function tests and creatine phosphokinase (CPK) in order to detect any possible adverse side-effects

CHD 9. Antiplatelet therapy. *The percentage of patients with CHD with a record in the last 15 months that aspirin, an alternative antiplatelet therapy, or an anticoagulant is being taken (unless a contraindication or side-effects are recorded) (7 points). (Minimum threshold = 25%, Maximum threshold = 90%.)*

It is anticipated that many patients with CHD will already be on prophylactic treatment with aspirin, an alternative antiplatelet therapy or an anticoagulant such as warfarin. Where this is not the case, it is important to arrange a consultation with the patient and prescribe appropriately if there is no contraindication. One could then start them on low-dose aspirin therapy subject to their agreement as well as providing an explanation as to its benefits and so advocating evidence-based medicine (EBM).

CHD 10. Beta blocker. *The percentage of patients with CHD who are currently treated with a beta blocker (unless a contraindication or side-effects are recorded) (7 points). (Minimum threshold = 25%, Maximum threshold = 50%.)*

This is a particularly difficult target to achieve as some clinicians only prescribe beta blockers following a myocardial infarction (MI) where they have been demonstrated in the literature to reduce mortality by up to a quarter and reinfarction by two-thirds or where there is angina. A dilemma arises whether to prescribe these drugs in somebody who has CHD, but not hypertension, angina or a recent MI. This is an area of the new contract where there is debate over the evidence base. The benefits of beta blockers in patients with angina or following an MI appear to have been extended to all patients with CHD.

Perhaps this is why the target levels for this indicator have been set lower with a maximum threshold of 50%, unlike most of the other indicators. Following a myocardial infarction patients should ideally be initiated and continued on a beta blocker on an indefinite basis. Where there are no contraindications and patients can tolerate the side-effects, beta blockers should be considered if they are not already taking them. They may also be given with ACE inhibitors as their effect in reducing mortality is thought to be cumulative.

For those patients in whom there is any contraindication, e.g., a patient with asthma or if they suffer side-effects, then it may be possible to absent these patients from the required quality indicator target through exception reporting and the mechanism for this will be discussed later.

CHD 11. Myocardial infarction and ACE inhibitor therapy. *The percentage of patients with a history of an MI (diagnosed after 1 April 2003) who are currently treated with an ACE inhibitor (7 points). (Minimum threshold = 25%, Maximum threshold = 70%.)*

It is now well recognised that this group of drugs as well as beta blockers can reduce mortality in patients who have suffered an MI and it is important to advise this therapy at review. For patients who are not able to tolerate an ACE inhibitor – for example, if they developed an ACE inhibitor cough – an angiotension II antagonist (A2) may be substituted for the purposes of the new contract. In relation to CHD indicator 10 above, ACE inhibitors have been proven to be beneficial in all patients with CHD, whether or not they have suffered an MI.

Practical point
Indicators CHD 10 and CHD 11 may cause some clinicians concern and judgements need to be made on an individual patient basis and if appropriate specialist advice should be sought.

CHD 12. Influenza vaccination. *The percentage of patients with CHD who have a record of influenza vaccination in the preceding 1 September to 31 March (7 points.) (Minimum threshold = 25%, Maximum threshold = 85%.)*

This is another common quality indicator that appears in five of the chronic diseases of the clinical domain of the QOF. It is therefore important for both health promotion and gaining points through the new contract to ensure that all high-risk patients – for example, those with CHD – are immunised against influenza. This will hopefully prevent any exacerbation of their current medical condition through an influenza infection.

Practical point
Further income may be gained through the profits associated with dispensing and the bulk purchase of influenza vaccines at a discounted cost to the practice. Influenza vaccination is also one of the Directed Enhanced Services for which there is a further payment for at-risk patients and those over 65 years of age.

Subset: Left Ventricular Dysfunction (LVD) (heart failure)

In terms of the new contract, many GPs are aware that heart failure is an important aspect. In relation to the quality indicators, it is a subset category of CHD and referred to as left ventricular dysfunction (LVD). In clinical practice, LVD may be at a very early stage and may not have presented with clinical symptoms and signs. However, in addition to patients who have subclinical LVD those who are at high risk of LVD include those who have had a myocardial infarction, patients who have hypertension or atrial fibrillation, but there are many other causes too.

Heart failure is a progressive disorder and one that results from damage to the heart. If it is detected and treated early, there may be a reduction in both morbidity and mortality. It can be picked up as a result of clinical suspicion or through investigations such as a chest x-ray where the heart size is reported as being greater than normal limits or through an abnormal electrocadiogram (ECG). In order to verify the diagnosis of heart failure the new GP contract requires that each patient diagnosed after 1 April 2003 has an echocardiogram (ECHO) performed. It is anticipated that through improved treatment of heart failure the hospital admission rate for the condition will be reduced and so will mortality. The reason that heart failure has been put as a subset of CHD is that CHD is the commonest cause of heart failure in the Western world.

In relation to the new contract, heart failure has been given particular recognition because it is an increasingly common problem in the population with increasing longevity. Some estimates have been made that this condition may result in 2% of the use of hospital beds and it has been predicted that there could be a 50% increase in the number of emergency admissions due to heart failure over the next 25 years. There are three quality indicators of heart failure with a total of 20 quality points as follows.

LVD 1. Disease register. *The practice is able to produce a register of patients with CHD and left ventricular dysfunction (4 points).*

Many of the patients who will be placed in this register can be identified from the repeat prescribing programme. For those patients diagnosed before April 2003, different criteria may have been used to make the diagnosis of heart failure and this diagnosis will be acceptable for this quality indicator under the new contract. However, as discussed earlier this will not be the case for diagnoses made after 1 April 2003. It is therefore recommended that patients with suspected heart failure are not Read coded until an ECHO has been performed as detailed in LVD 2.

LVD 2. LVD confirmed by an ECHO. The percentage of patients with a diagnosis of CHD and left ventricular dysfunction (diagnosed after 1 April 2003) should be recorded who have had their diagnosis confirmed by an ECHO (6 points). (Minimum threshold = 25%, Maximum threshold = 90%.)

An ECHO is an absolute method to verify the diagnosis of heart failure. Many NHS trusts are offering a rapid service for ECHOs to enable GPs to set up their heart failure registers and promote appropriate treatment and regular review of this group of patients.

LVD 3. Treatment with ACE inhibitors (or A2 antagonists). *The percentage of patients with a diagnosis of CHD and left ventricular dysfunction who are currently treated with ACE inhibitors (or A2 antagonists) (10 points). (Minimum threshold = 25%, Maximum threshold = 70%.)*

A drug of choice for the treatment of heart failure is an ACE inhibitor and the number of points available for this quality indicator support this clinical statement. However, it is possible to exempt patients where this medication is contraindicated such as aortic or renal artery stenosis or severe renal impairment. If medication is started in this group then they should be closely monitored and started with the lowest dose of the individual drug chosen and the dose titrated accordingly with clinical response.

Total points available for CHD = 121

> **Practical point**
> There are ten chronic diseases within the clinical domain of the QOF and there are two ways of collecting the necessary data, ordering investigations and advising regarding particular medications in order that quality indicator points may be claimed. These are:
> - opportunistically during a routine consultation
> - organised recall and review using a disease register.
>
> When reviewing patients with any of the ten chronic diseases of the clinical domain of the QOF, it is important to be aware of any of the other nine conditions that can be discussed and reviewed at the same time. In order to facilitate this activity, the practice computer system must have the necessary templates which are correctly Read coded.

Opportunistic chronic disease care during a routine consultation

All GPs are busy and this process should be made as easy and user-friendly as possible and the opportunistic way is perhaps the most important. Take the example of a patient with diabetes who defaults hospital clinics and also the GP diabetes clinic. When that person consults for another reason is maybe the only opportunity to devote some of the limited consultation time in relation to their diabetes. Therefore an easily accessible diabetes computer template should be available to the doctor or the practice nurse so that they can see at a glance which quality indicators are required to be fulfilled.

> **Practical point**
> For those doctors who do not like using computers in the consultation or find them cumbersome, the practice manager should provide a handwritten format of the template, which the doctor completes during or at the end of the consultation. The doctor should then pass the information to the practice manager so that it may be entered on the appropriate template of the practice computer system.

Stroke

Cerebrovascular accidents (CVAs)/strokes are common and are the major cause of severe disability in the UK. Risk factors include hypertension, atrial fibrillation, raised cholesterol, smoking and diabetes. In addition, those patients who have suffered a transient ischaemic attack (TIA) or who have had a previous stroke are at particular risk. It is thought that up to 100 000 people in England and Wales have a stroke each year. It is for this reason that the new contract includes stroke as one of the ten chronic diseases within the clinical domain. Several of the other chronic diseases that also appear within the clinical domain of the new contract – for example, hypertension – are aimed at preventing both strokes and CHD.

There are ten separate quality indicators with the abbreviation STROKE with a total of 31 points.

Records

STROKE 1. Disease register. *The practice can produce a register of patients with stroke and TIA (4 points).*

Every practice will be able to perform a computer search to identify many of the patients who have suffered with a stroke or TIA in order to create this register. In addition, individual doctors will be able to name patients known to them who have suffered a stroke, particularly those who are severely disabled as a result and require regular medical review.

For patients who were diagnosed with these conditions prior to April 2003, the diagnosis will be accepted for the purposes of the register. However, after this date it is important that patients are not entered onto the register until it has been confirmed with diagnostic radiological imaging as detailed below.

STROKE 2. Confirmation by CT or MRI scan. *The percentage of new patients with presumptive stroke (presenting after 1 April 2003) who have been referred for confirmation of the diagnosis by CT or MRI scan (2 points). (Minimum threshold = 25%, Maximum threshold = 80%.)*

This may be a difficult target to achieve given waiting list times for these investigations. Therefore, if a patient develops signs of a possible stroke they may require hospital admission in order to make the diagnosis by Computerised (Axial) Tomography (CT) scan or Magnetic Resonance Imaging (MRI) scan. The Scottish Intercollegiate Guidelines Network (SIGN) guideline number 13 states that these investigations should be performed within 48 hours of the development of symptoms. It may also be that some practices have the availability of a fast-track clinic for this condition.

Practical point
Although it is not essential under the new contract for people who have had a TIA to have these scans, it may be very helpful in their medical management to ascertain the cause, for example, vascular or non-vascular.

Ongoing management

STROKE 3. Smoking status. *The percentage of patients with TIA or stroke who have a record of smoking status in the last 15 months, except those who have never smoked where smoking status should be recorded at least once since diagnosis (3 points). (Minimum threshold = 25%, Maximum threshold = 90%.)*

It is important to ascertain the number of TIA or stroke patients who smoke so that they can be targeted for smoking cessation advice and so hopefully reduce further events.

STROKE 4. Smoking cessation advice. *The percentage of patients with a history of TIA or stroke who smoke and whose notes contain a record that smoking cessation advice has been offered in the last 15 months (2 points). (Minimum threshold = 25%, Maximum threshold = 70%.)*

As has been stated previously there are several chronic disease conditions where it is good medical practice to advise patients to stop smoking and to provide the necessary service to enable them to do this.

Practical point
When this advice is given it must be recorded on the computer for all patients who are smokers.

STROKE 5. Blood pressure recording. *The percentage of patients with TIA or stroke who have a record of blood pressure in the notes in the preceding 15 months (2 points). (Minimum threshold = 25%, Maximum threshold = 90%.)*

It is important that stroke and TIA patients are followed up and a very important part of their review is blood pressure measurement.

STROKE 6. Blood pressure 150/90 or less. *The percentage of patients with a history of TIA or stroke in whom the last blood pressure reading (measured in the last 15 months) is 150/90 or less (5 points). (Minimum threshold = 25%, Maximum threshold = 70%.)*

It is anticipated that the lower a patient's blood pressure is following a stroke or TIA, the less chance they have of recurrence. It therefore seems reasonable to be aggressive in ensuring that their blood pressure measurements are 150/90 or less through lifestyle advice and appropriate medication if it is required.

STROKE 7. Cholesterol. *The percentage of patients with TIA or stroke who have a record of total cholesterol in the last 15 months (2 points). (Minimum threshold = 25%, Maximum threshold = 90%.)*

The disability suffered as the result of a stroke is often irreversible and any interventions that can be made to reduce the possibility of further stroke should be undertaken. Therefore, as part of an annual review of patients who have had a history of TIA or stroke, the measurement of cholesterol and associated lipids is important.

STROKE 8. Cholesterol 5 or less. *The percentage of patients with TIA or stroke whose last measured total cholesterol (measured in the last 15 months) is 5 mmol/l or less (5 points). (Minimum threshold = 25%, Maximum threshold = 60%.)*

For those patients who have suffered a TIA or a stroke it is important to offer medication if their cholesterol remains above 5 despite appropriate dietary measures.

STROKE 9. Antiplatelet therapy. *The percentage of patients with a stroke shown to be non-haemorrhagic, or a history of TIA, who have a record that aspirin, an alternative antiplatelet therapy, or an anticoagulant is being taken (unless a contraindication or side-effects are recorded) (4 points). (Minimum threshold = 25%, Maximum threshold – 90%.)*

Long-term antiplatelet therapy can reduce the risk of further vascular events for those who have had a non-haemorrhagic TIA or stroke. It is important, therefore, that patients are informed of the medication that is available and are invited to be part of the decision-making process as to which medication is prescribed.

STROKE 10. Influenza immunisation. *The percentage of patients with TIA or stroke who have had influenza immunisation in the preceding 1 September to 31 March (2 points). (Minimum threshold = 25%, Maximum threshold = 85%.)*

Patients who have suffered a stroke may have associated disability and if they are to get an influenza infection this is likely to exacerbate the disability for some considerable time. In addition there will be a risk of increased mortality. It is important therefore to advise such patients of the benefits of influenza vaccination where there are no contraindications. For patients who are severely disabled vaccination at home may be required.

Total points available for patients with Stroke or a TIA = 31

In large practices, it may be decided to set up a stroke clinic in order to review patients annually and so gain the necessary points for the ten quality indicators that had been listed. For patients who are severely disabled as a result of a stroke there will be informal carers and this is an opportunity to find out their healthcare needs and whether they are coping. This will also help to create part of the register of informal carers which is the ninth quality indicator of the fourth organisational domain – practice management.

Practical point
How is the practice performing? In order to inform recall from disease registers and to identify patients who are defaulting from review consultations or clinics, it is important to have a programme on the practice GP computer software which allows a monthly audit of performance in each of the ten chronic diseases. In our practice, we have a programme called 'Population Manager', which enables this process to happen rather than waiting for the PCO audit in March 2005 when it could be too late. The new contract by its very nature is proactive rather than reactive and so promoting health in those with chronic disease.

Hypertension

Hypertension is a common medical problem which is detected by screening and is often asymptomatic. However, it is a significant factor in other serious conditions including coronary heart disease, cerebrovascular disease and diabetes. The incidence of hypertension increases with age and may affect up to half of the population over the age of 65 years. There has been much recent debate in the literature as to the levels at which hypertension can be defined, but for the purpose of the new contract targets for blood pressure are stated as 150/90 or below and 145/85 or below for diabetes.

At first glance it might be thought that hypertension does not figure prominently as a chronic disease of the clinical domain of the QOF as there are only five quality indicators. However, the total number of points available for quality care in hypertension is exactly one-tenth of the total number of points that are available. The proportion is higher still when the other three chronic diseases that have quality indicators for hypertension are included. In order to achieve these points, considerable emphasis is placed on regularly measuring the blood pressure of patients with hypertension and at least once every nine months.

Approximately half of the points are for ensuring that patients on the disease register for hypertension have a blood pressure of 150/90 or less. So in addition to measuring the blood pressure of a patient with hypertension it is important to ensure that treatment with advice or medication reduces their blood pressure to a reading of 150/90 or less and 145/85 or less in patients with diabetes.

First and most important is the need to set up the disease register which will be a large register in any practice given the extent of hypertension in the general population. For practices already using computers this register is likely to be well established and it is easy to search for common hypertension medications to discover those patients that are not on the hypertension register but should be. Care needs to be taken with medications such as propranolol where the indication may be for anxiety and ACE inhibitors which may be being used to treat heart failure. It is important therefore when establishing the complete register that each possible entry onto the register is correct. In addition, there will be a few patients who have hypertension, particularly borderline hypertension, who are not on any medication.

Practical point
Ideal repeat prescribing programmes will have a link where the clinical reason for each medication can be identified.

There are five separate quality indicators, with the abbreviation BP for Blood Pressure, with a total of 105 points.

Records

BP 1. Disease register. *The practice can produce a register of patients with established hypertension (9 points).*

This is likely to be a large register given the extent of hypertension in the general population.

Diagnosis and initial management

BP 2. Smoking status. *The percentage of patients with hypertension whose notes record smoking status at least once (10 points). (Minimum threshold = 25%, Maximum threshold = 90%.)*

Smoking status features in several of the chronic diseases of the clinical domain of the QOF and this information is easy to record and easy to obtain from patients opportunistically.

BP 3. Smoking cessation advice. *The percentage of patients with hypertension who smoke, whose notes contain a record that smoking cessation advice has been offered at least once (10 points). (Minimum threshold = 25%, Maximum threshold = 90%.)*

As detailed previously, smoking cessation advice should always be recorded. This advice is important for the future health of smokers and hypertension is no exception.

Ongoing management

BP 4. Blood pressure measurement. *The percentage of patients with hypertension in which there is a record of the blood pressure in the past nine months (20 points). (Minimum threshold = 25%, Maximum threshold = 90%.)*

To ensure that 90% of patients with hypertension have their blood pressure measured every nine months is a difficult target to achieve. Their blood pressure can be measured opportunistically when they consult for a reason other than hypertension or they can be recalled by performing a computer search to find out which patients with hypertension have not had their blood pressure measured in the last nine months. For those patients with hypertension who are on medication and therefore on the repeat prescribing programme, the practice computer system can be used to alert the doctor at six months to say that a patient has not had their blood pressure measured. A reminder note can then be placed on their repeat prescription to ask them to attend the surgery for a measurement.

BP 5. Blood pressure 150/90 or less. *The percentage of patients with hypertension in whom the last blood pressure (measured in last nine months) is 150/90 or less (56 points). (Minimum threshold = 25%, Maximum threshold = 70%.)*

It is difficult enough to measure the blood pressure of every patient with hypertension in the preceding nine months, but to obtain a reading that is 150/90 or less must surely be a considerable challenge for 70% of the population in the practice who have hypertension. Those patients whose blood pressure is not satisfactorily controlled will need to be encouraged to attend the practice regularly and be willing to both change medication and/or take additional medication until their blood pressure is brought under control as defined by the new contract.

Although hypertension is the basis for a common consultation, to achieve this particularly high number of points for this chronic disease in the QOF requires a lot of work on behalf of the practice team. However, its potential benefits in reducing morbidity and mortality will be considerable to practices.

Practical point
56 points are available for this single quality indicator and this should be brought to the attention of all members of the PHCT.

It may seem a small point, but it is important to ensure in overweight patients that their blood pressure has been measured with an appropriate size cuff rather than a standard size cuff. In addition, some patients may be able to monitor their own blood pressure if they purchase the necessary equipment and this may help to reduce the issue of 'white coat hypertension' and empower patients to take responsibility for their own health and management of disease conditions such as hypertension. *See* Stergiou G *et al.* (2004) Self-monitoring of blood pressure at home (editorial). *BMJ.* **329**: 870–1.

Total points available for Hypertension = 105

Practical point

Hypertension is a good example of planning the practice workforce. In order to attain optimal blood pressure control, patients will need to be reviewed regularly, but this may not be a good use of the doctor's time. Such work may be delegated to other members of the team; for example, a Health Care Assistant (HCA) working to a strict practice protocol may be employed to help in the review process to achieve these difficult targets. Also the use of a phlebotomist for appropriate blood tests taken at the time hypertension is suspected and indicated by the initiation of particular antihypertensives will be helpful.

Success in achieving quality indicator targets requires a lot of hard work and close working by all of the team members.

Diabetes

There are 18 separate quality indicators, with the abbreviation DM for Diabetes, with a total of 99 points. With the designation of these 99 (almost 10%) of the target or indicator points, diabetes is another one of the important contributors to the QOF. To attain all 99 points will require good clinical and organisational skills.

Why is diabetes attributed such importance? Diabetes types I and II are major independent risk factors for coronary artery disease and death rates from heart disease in this group of people are two to four times higher than people who do not have diabetes. In addition, diabetes is also associated with generalised macrovascular and microvascular disease and so complications that may affect the eyes, kidneys and the circulation to the lower limbs. In addition, diabetes adversely affects those who are pregnant. Furthermore, diabetes is a common condition and the prevalence of diabetes is increasing which is a global trend, not just in the UK. It impacts considerably on quality of life and healthcare planning and resources.

Records

DM 1. Disease register. *The practice can produce a register of all patients with diabetes mellitus (6 points).*

A register is vital to enable recall and performing an annual review. Please refer to the 'Blue Book' previously detailed for the criteria by which the diagnosis of diabetes can be made, e.g., how the diagnosis is made from random, fasting glucoses and glucose tolerance tests. As with all diseases it is important to record the date of diagnosis and the blood tests performed at the time to verify the diagnosis.

Ongoing management

DM 2. Body mass index. *The percentage of patients with diabetes whose notes record body mass index (BMI) in the previous 15 months (3 points). (Minimum threshold = 25%, Maximum threshold = 90%.)*

Ultimately, this will mean ensuring that all patients on the register have been weighed in the proceeding 15 months as it is anticipated that the height should already be recorded and should be relatively static in adults. Children and adolescents with diabetes should have their height checked – also perhaps patients with known osteoporosis with documented vertebral collapse who may have a significant loss in their height.

DM 3. Smoking status. *The percentage of patients with diabetes in whom there is a record of smoking status in the previous 15 months except those who have never smoked where smoking status should be recorded once (3 points). (Minimum threshold = 25%, Maximum threshold = 90%.)*

As stated earlier recording smoking status is important and diabetes is no exception.

DM 4. Smoking cessation advice. *The percentage of patients with diabetes who smoke and whose notes contain a record that smoking cessation advice has been offered in the last 15 months (5 points). (Minimum threshold = 25%, Maximum threshold = 90%.)*

For people with diabetes who smoke, smoking is yet a further risk factor for CHD and other diseases, and patients should be given cessation advice and this information recorded with the appropriate Read code.

DM 5. Glycosylated haemoglobin (HbA1c). *The percentage of patients with diabetes who have a record of HbA1c or equivalent in the previous 15 months (3 points). (Minimum threshold = 25%, Maximum threshold = 90%.)*

This is an important measure of overall diabetes control that is necessary to assess the progress of patients with diabetes. This is additional information to a diary of blood glucoses and fasting glucoses that may have been recorded.

DM 6. Glycosylated haemoglobin (HbA1c) < 7.4%. *The percentage of patients with diabetes in whom the last HbA1c is 7.4 or less (or equivalent test/reference range depending on local laboratory) in last 15 months (16 points). (Minimum threshold = 25%, Maximum threshold = 50%.)*

At first sight this might seem a particularly difficult target to attain, but the maximum threshold is 50%, rather than 90%. Therefore half of the practice's patients on the diabetes register need an HbA1c of 7.4% or less. This will involve close working and so shared care with colleagues in secondary care both in the collection of the data and agreed management plans. In addition, close attention to patients who default clinic follow-up will be required. NICE guidelines (September 2002) state that a target HbA1c should be between 6.5% and 7.5%, based on the risk of vascular complications. It is important to take care with patients who are prone to hypoglycaemia, particularly those who get limited or no early warning of hypoglycaemia and so to be cautious when increasing medication. Overall this is not an easy target to achieve given that all diabetes services will care for a mixed population of individuals with diabetes. The next indicator, DM 7, is somewhat easier to achieve and has a reward of a significant number of points.

DM 7. Glycosylated haemoglobin (HbA1c) < 10%. *The percentage of patients with diabetes in whom the last HbA1c is 10% or less (or equivalent test/reference range depending on local laboratory) in last 15 months (11 points). (Minimum threshold = 25%, Maximum threshold = 85%.)*

For those patients with type II diabetes and an HbA1c of 10% or greater, urgent review is required, and where control is difficult to achieve, therapy with insulin may need to be considered.

DM 8. Retinal screening. *The percentage of patients with diabetes who have a record of retinal screening in the previous 15 months (5 points). (Minimum threshold = 25%, Maximum threshold = 90%.)*

Retinal screening may be undertaken by the GP, local approved optician or by the hospital clinic. It is important that correspondence is carefully read and screening documented under the correct Read code.

DM 9. Peripheral pulses. *The percentage of patients with diabetes with a record of presence or absence of peripheral pulses in the previous 15 months (3 points). (Minimum threshold = 25%, Maximum threshold = 90%.)*

Like all of the indicators patients with diabetes need to be seen each year at the GP or hospital clinic and a recall system put in place to follow up those who default clinic attendance. This is good preventive medicine as these are likely to be the patients most at risk of complications.

DM 10. Neuropathy. *The percentage of patients with diabetes with a record of neuropathy testing in the previous 15 months (3 points). (Minimum threshold = 25%, Maximum threshold = 90%.)*

Neuropathy is a generic phrase relating to functional disturbances or pathological changes in the peripheral nervous system. If the involvement is in one nerve this is referred to as mononeuropathy, if involvement is several nerves this is referred to as mononeuritis multiplex, and if is diffuse and bilateral this is referred to as poly-neuropathy. The symptoms of peripheral neuropathy vary but usually start with numbness, pain or weakness – for example, sensory disturbance, pins and needles, burning sensations and muscle weakness. Diabetes is one of the most common known causes of peripheral neuropathy and may affect 10% or more of people with diabetes. The development of neuropathy may be slowed down by close control of a person's diabetes. Why is neuropathy of concern? Numb skin needs to be protected from injury as small bumps and knocks may not be felt and can rapidly turn into infected ulcers that are slow to heal. Also irritated nerves can cause pain and burning and so be unpleasant and there are medications which may alleviate these symptoms.

DM 11.   Blood pressure. The percentage of patients with diabetes who have a record of the blood pressure in the past 15 months (3 points). (Minimum threshold = 25%, Maximum threshold = 90%.)

As detailed under Hypertension, it is important that patients with diabetes have their blood pressure measured regularly as they are at a greater risk of hypertension and CHD.

DM 12. Blood pressure 145/85 or less. *The percentage of patients with diabetes in whom the last blood pressure is 145/85 or less (17 points). (Minimum threshold = 25%, Maximum threshold = 55%.)*

This is another difficult target to achieve with nearly 20% of the available points to claim for diabetes. It indicates the importance of good blood pressure control attributed to patients with diabetes and perhaps this target is more realistically defined where the maximum threshold is 55%.

DM 13. Microalbuminuria testing. *The percentage of patients with diabetes who have a record of microalbuminuria testing in the previous 15 months. Patients with proteinuria can have exception reporting (3 points). (Minimum threshold = 25%, Maximum threshold = 90%.)*

Testing stix are available to detect the presence of microalbuminuria or local hospital laboratories may be able to undertake this testing. Exception reporting is possible for patients with existing proteinuria and this must be coded separately as detailed at the end of the chapter.

DM 14. Creatinine. *The percentage of patients with diabetes who have a record of serum creatinine testing in the previous 15 months (3 points). (Minimum threshold = 25%, Maximum threshold = 90%.)*

For patients with microalbuminuria or proteinuria or under-diagnosed nephropathy this is an important parameter of renal function to measure.

DM 15. Proteinuria or microalbuminuria treated with ACE inhibitors (or A2 antagonists). *The percentage of patients with diabetes with proteinuria or microalbuminuria who are treated with ACE inhibitors (or A2 antagonists) (3 points). (Minimum threshold = 25%, Maximum threshold = 70%.)*

Good practice is recognised in relation to the treatment of patients with diabetes who have microalbuminuria or proteinuria and so early renal impairment. It is important that they receive appropriate treatment with ACE inhibitors or A2 antagonists which will also help to control co-existing hypertension and assist in meeting the DM 12 indicator. Exception reporting is possible for patients in whom ACE inhibitors (or A2 antagonists) are contraindicated.

DM 16. Cholesterol. *The percentage of patients with diabetes who have a record of total cholesterol in the previous 15 months (3 points). (Minimum threshold = 25%, Maximum threshold = 90%.)*

Raised cholesterol is being increasingly recognised as a further risk factor in patients with diabetes and it is important that it is measured on at least an annual basis.

DM 17. Cholesterol is 5 or less. *The percentage of patients with diabetes whose last measured total cholesterol within previous 15 months is 5 or less (6 points). (Minimum threshold = 25%, Maximum threshold = 60%.)*

Patients who do not have a cholesterol of 5 or less should be considered for treatment with statins and provided with further dietary advice as appropriate.

Practical point

Prescribing costs for an individual practice may rise significantly in several areas as a result of the implementation of the QOF, e.g., the use of statins to lower serum cholesterol levels. PCOs may or may not take this into account in individual regions in relation to possible 'prescribing incentives'.

DM 18. Influenza vaccination. *The percentage of patients with diabetes who have had influenza immunisation in the preceding months (1 September to 31 March) (3 points). (Minimum threshold = 25%, Maximum threshold = 85%.)*

As the maximum threshold is set at 85% for influenza vaccination this allows 15% of patients to decline or who have had a previous adverse reaction to vaccination.

Total points available for Diabetes = 99

Chronic Obstructive Pulmonary Disease (COPD)

In clinical practice, it is important to make a distinction between the two chronic conditions of asthma and COPD. This is because their medical management is different. The two conditions can be distinguished by spirometry and the use of reversibility testing to diagnose COPD. Asthma results in reversible airways obstruction whereas in COPD the reversibility of the airways obstruction is reduced with increasing severity of the disease. (Please see under COPD 3 and the recent controversy and debate in relation to NICE guidelines and reversibility testing.) COPD may be defined as airflow obstruction that is usually progressive, not fully reversible and does not change markedly over several months. The disease is predominantly caused by smoking.

In order to achieve the quality indicators that relate to COPD, a practice needs to consider whether a separate clinic is created to perform spirometry and reversibility testing. This will depend on the size of a practice, the number of patients suspected to suffer with COPD and if there is a practice nurse who would like to develop specialist interest in this condition. In addition, it will be necessary for the practice to invest in a spirometer.

The reason that COPD has such prominence within the new contract is because it is a condition that can lead to considerable morbidity and premature death. It is a condition that is under-diagnosed and it may be mistaken as a person suffering with recurrent chest infections, particularly in smokers. It may not be recognised until a person has lost a considerable proportion of their respiratory function. With the development of new treatments, it is therefore important to make the diagnosis. Also for those people where the condition is advanced, it is important to provide symptomatic treatment and so try and maintain a patient's quality of life. In some centres, e.g. Oxford, a pulmonary rehabilitation programme is available to increase exercise tolerance. A further reason for early diagnosis is to advise the patient who is smoking to stop through a smoking cessation clinic as those who continue to smoke will decline by more than twice as much per year compared to those who have stopped smoking. (Price D and Duerden M (2003) Editorial: COPD. *BMJ.* **326:** 1046–7.)

There are eight separate quality indicators, with the abbreviation COPD for Chronic Obstructive Pulmonary Disease, with a total of 45 points.

Records

COPD 1. Disease register. *The practice can produce a register of patients with COPD (5 points). Existing patients may be obtained from computer search and by questioning the individual doctors.*

If a search is made under inhaled medication it will be necessary to differentiate between asthma and COPD. It may also be useful to search under the term emphysema as some of these patients may be COPD patients. For patients who are newly diagnosed with COPD the exact diagnosis will require to be confirmed by spirometry.

Initial diagnosis

COPD 2. Spirometry. *The percentage of patients where the diagnosis has been confirmed by spirometry including reversibility testing for newly diagnosed patients with effect from 1 April 2003 (5 points). (Minimum threshold = 25%, Maximum threshold = 90%.)*

Where a practice does not possess its own spirometer then it will be necessary to make a referral to a local secondary care unit where the necessary testing can be undertaken. However, it should be borne in mind that there may be a waiting list for this service.

COPD 3. Spirometry including reversibility testing. *The percentage of all patients with COPD where diagnosis has been confirmed by spirometry including reversibility testing (5 points). (Minimum threshold = 25%, Maximum threshold = 90%.)*

This is an extension of the last quality indicator and includes all patients with COPD prior to 1 April 2003. This quality indicator has caused some recent controversy as NICE guidelines published earlier in 2004 suggested that reversibility testing was of no benefit. The main reason for this is that reversibility testing is inconsistent and so can be difficult to reproduce and it does not necessarily predict response to bronchodilators or inhaled corticosteroids. Reversibility testing with bronchodilators and/or oral steroids can however be useful to try and distinguish between asthma and COPD. The other area of controversy in relation to this quality indicator is that the previous gold standard of the British Thoracic Society (BTS) is where the guideline is a reduced post-bronchodilator forced expiratory volume in one second (FEV1) < 80% predicted. In the new contract the level is set at FEV1 < 70% predicted. It is hoped that revised guidelines will be made in the not too distant future regarding this although it could be argued that this figure will concentrate attention on patients in whom one would expect to have symptoms.

Ongoing management

COPD 4. Smoking status. *The percentage of patients with COPD in whom there is a record of smoking status in the previous 15 months (6 points). (Minimum threshold = 25%, Maximum threshold = 90%.)*

Again, the importance of asking whether a patient smokes or not is a recurrent theme in the QOF and as detailed above is vital information in relation to the aetiology and natural history of COPD.

COPD 5. Smoking cessation advice. *The percentage of patients with COPD who smoke, whose notes contain a record that smoking cessation advice has been offered in the past 15 months (6 points). (Minimum threshold = 25%, Maximum threshold = 90%.)*

It makes good clinical sense to offer patients with COPD smoking cessation advice to try and slow the progression of their condition as this intervention has been shown to dramatically slow the rate of COPD progression. This is because the disease is predominantly caused by smoking, although certain occupations also predispose to the development of the condition. In addition, significant airflow obstruction may be present before a person is aware of it.

COPD 6. FEV1. *The percentage of patients with COPD with a record of FEV1 in the previous 27 months (6 points). (Minimum threshold = 25%, Maximum threshold = 70%.)*

In order to gain an FEV1 reading, the practice will require a spirometer or access to a specialist service. As well as entering the Read code (68M) for FEV1 it is useful to record the numerical value so that it is possible to monitor patients and so identify those who may require oxygen therapy in the future. An FEV1 reading is the percentage of the total lung volume that can be forcibly exhaled in one second from maximum inspiration. This decreases with age, and in those people who have obstructive airways disease, which may be asthma or COPD, the reading may be less than 70%.

COPD 7. Inhaler technique. *The percentage of patients with COPD receiving inhaled treatment in whom there is a record that inhaler technique has been checked in the preceding two years (6 points). (Minimum threshold = 25%, Maximum threshold = 90%.)*

Patients will not gain optimal benefit from inhaled medication if their inhaler technique is poor and it would be appropriate to check this at annual review and provide advice as necessary.

COPD 8. Influenza vaccination. *The percentage of patients with COPD who have had influenza immunisation in the preceding 1 September to 31 March (6 points). (Minimum threshold = 25%, Maximum threshold = 85%.)*

Influenza is particularly detrimental in people with COPD as it is likely to lead to a chest infection and if vaccination is not contraindicated it should be strongly advocated. Similarly, it would be appropriate in this particular group of patients to check that they have had a pneumococcal vaccine in the last ten years. This is not part of the new contract, but is good clinical practice.

Total points available for COPD = 45

The importance of differentiating asthma from COPD

It is important to differentiate asthma from COPD. The management of COPD requires the application of several therapies at the same time in an integrated way. However, asthma requires a stepwise approach until control is achieved and maintained. Asthma is not usually a progressive condition and so does not require further medication in an increasing dose regime in order to maintain control. COPD and the new contract as detailed above has shown some discrepancies with national guidelines. However, these are likely to be revised in future. In the meantime, the most important aspect of the chronic disease of COPD is creating a register that can be used to audit this group of patients. This will inevitably make one reconsider the diagnostic criteria that have perhaps previously been used for asthma and so detect those patients who have been labelled as having asthma, but who in fact have COPD. As a result this will help practices to earn quality points for asthma care which is discussed later.

Practical point
COPD is a condition where some patients may be housebound. In relation to all the quality indicators it is important for each practice to develop an effective way of following up and managing housebound patients. In relation to the quality indicators there are no extra funds for visiting patients at home and, where appropriate, delegation to other members of the team may be necessary to ensure these patients are adequately cared for. It is likely that these patients will be at the end stage of their chronic disease and so both the patient and their carer will be in need of healthcare input. In turn, this activity will be rewarded through the attainment of quality indicator points.

Epilepsy

Epilepsy is a common neurological condition in practice and one that can be associated with a high morbidity and so have a severe impact on a person's quality of life. Epilepsy is where there is abnormal electrical activity in the brain which can lead an individual to suffer repeated seizures (convulsions) and possible loss of consciousness. In those patients where epilepsy is not adequately controlled there is also an increase in mortality.

It is estimated that nearly half a million people in the UK have epilepsy. The type and frequency of seizures differs between individuals and it is believed that up to 70% of those with epilepsy should be able to be seizure free on the correct medication. The new contract will promote practices to create a disease register for patients with epilepsy and so a basis for regular review. It is recommended that for patients on this register the following information should be recorded in their records:

- type of seizures together with frequency and date of last seizure
- medication – type and dose being prescribed
- any adverse reactions to medication for epilepsy
- review and care plan.

There are four separate quality indicators for epilepsy with a total of 16 points.

Records

EPILEPSY 1. Disease register. *The practice can produce a register of patients receiving drug treatment for epilepsy (2 points).*

The register is therefore people who currently suffer with epilepsy, and not individuals who have been treated for epilepsy in the past but have been seizure free since stopping medication. In order to create an epilepsy disease register it is important to search under common drugs that are used to treat epilepsy. However, it should not be assumed that all anticonvulsants are being prescribed for epilepsy. For example, carbamazepine is sometimes used in the control of neuropathic pain. It is therefore important to examine the medical records to be sure the person has epilepsy, when it was diagnosed and what investigations were performed at the time of diagnosis. One could expect the Practice Prevalence for this condition to be somewhere between five and ten cases per thousand patients.

Ongoing management

EPILEPSY 2. Seizure frequency. *The percentage of patients age 16 and over on drug treatment for epilepsy who have a record of seizure frequency in the previous 15 months (4 points). (Minimum threshold = 25%, Maximum threshold = 90%.)*

In order to meet this quality indicator, the disease register should be used as a basis for annual recall and so review of patients aged 16 years or over who are taking anticonvulsant medication for epilepsy. At these review consultations it will be possible to determine seizure frequency including the date of the last seizure and whether their epilepsy is controlled. Where adequate control cannot be achieved referral to a specialist is indicated. Similarly, when patients do not respond to recall or fail to attend for your review, this is a reason for concern and repeated effort should be made to encourage such patients to attend.

Practical point
Children do not form part of the epilepsy quality indicators, but it is good clinical practice to record the same information for patients under the age of 16 years.

EPILEPSY 3. Medication review. *The percentage of patients age 16 and over on drug treatment for epilepsy who have a record of medication review in the previous 15 months (4 points). (Minimum threshold = 25%, Maximum threshold = 90%.)*

Annual reviews will also provide an opportunity to measure serum drug levels where this is indicated and if seizure control is not adequate, then the dose of medications may be adjusted. When undertaking a medication review it is important to ensure that drug side-effects are asked about. Other reasons for reviewing medication include patients who have been on long-term therapy and may be considering reducing and stopping their medication. This is something that can be discussed, carefully considered and negotiated as a recurrence of seizures will impact on activities of daily living and also driving. In order to ensure that annual review takes place, repeat prescription review dates should be no longer than a 12-month period.

EPILEPSY 4. Convulsion free for 12 months. *The percentage of patients age 16 and over on drug treatment for epilepsy who have been convulsion-free for last 12 months recorded in last 15 months (6 points). (Minimum threshold = 25%, Maximum threshold = 70%.)*

This information will be available if the patient is offered an annual review. This can be a difficult target to achieve and in some situations this may be the basis for exception reporting in patients where compliance with medication is difficult or where their epilepsy is a result of severe brain damage and it is not possible to achieve this optimal control of being convulsion free for a 12-month period.

If it is discovered that a patient is taking medication for epilepsy, but that the diagnosis has not been adequately confirmed by investigations such as an electro-encephalogram (EEG), then the issue of a misdiagnosis should be considered and shared with the patient. It will then be necessary to refer these patients to a specialist for appropriate investigations. Ideally, the diagnosis of epilepsy and initiation of anticonvulsant medication should only be made by a specialist. It has been suggested that the reason epilepsy has been included within the clinical domain of the QOF is that the care of epilepsy has until now been poorly recorded and sporadic. It seems strange therefore that only 16 points have been allocated to this condition.

When reviewing patients with epilepsy it is important to be aware of any other conditions that can be discussed at the same time: for example, a woman with epilepsy who wishes advice relating to possible pregnancy and the continued use of their medication – also, e.g., patients who have learning disabilities and whether other medical and social needs are being adequately met.

In relation to the 70% maximum threshold, the 'Blue Book' states, *'The top level of this indicator has been deliberately set at a lower level in order to encourage general practitioners to record the frequency of convulsions as accurately as possible.'* It is an opportunity to oversee a condition where improved recognition and clinical management will be beneficial to those who suffer with epilepsy on a practice list.

Total points available for Epilepsy = 16

Hypothyroidism

Hypothyroidism is a relatively common condition and may be a chance finding when routine blood tests are requested for symptoms such as tiredness. The definition of hypothyroidism would be where patients are receiving thyroxine replacement for proven hypothyroidism and not those patients who have borderline blood results (thyroid stimulating hormone – TSH), who are due to have this test repeated in the future.

Hypothyroidism is more common in females than males. The incidence in females is about 15 per 1000 of the population, whereas the incidence in males is about one per 1000 of the population. The diagnosis should be made biochemically where there is a reduction in free or total T4 with a rise in serum TSH using local laboratory references ranges. Where there is an elevated TSH with a normal serum T4 then the hypothyroidism is termed subclinical. If a clinician is in doubt about a diagnosis of hypothyroidism they should speak to a clinical biochemist. The measurement of serum free or total T3 is usually unhelpful, because T3 may be reduced only slightly as a result of increased peripheral conversion of T4 to T3.

There are two separate quality indicators, with the abbreviation THYROID for hypothyroidism, with a total of 8 points.

Records

THYROID 1. Disease register. *The practice can produce a register of patients with hypothyroidism (2 points).*

In those practices that are computerised, it should be straightforward to search for those patients who are taking thyroxine tablets. These patients can then be entered on the register. As with all diseases it is important to record the date of diagnosis and that blood tests were performed at the time to verify the diagnosis.

Ongoing management

THYROID 2. Thyroid function tests. *The percentage of patients with hypothyroidism with thyroid function tests (TFTs) recorded in the previous 15 months (6 points). (Minimum threshold = 25%, Maximum threshold = 90%.)*

It is important to review patients who are on long-term medication and patients taking thyroxine are no exception. If these patients are reviewed annually by performing a blood test for thyroid function tests (TFTs) two weeks prior to the review, then it is possible to inform patients whether they should continue taking the same dose of thyroxine.

Total points available for Hypothyroidism = 8

Cancer

Cancer is a common condition and a priority where care should be taken to follow people up. There are 38 Read codes covering the commoner malignancies. Some practices may keep a paper-based register of their patients with cancer and when creating a computer register it is important to use this information and also data entered on the computer where and when a patient has been diagnosed with cancer. It is important to code all new cases when correspondence from secondary care arrives with this information. Although most of cancer care takes place in secondary care the GP and the associated PHCT have a key role in co-ordinating the care of cancer patients.

There are two separate quality indicators denoted by CANCER with a total of 12 points.

Records

CANCER 1. Disease register. *The practice can produce a register of all cancer patients defined as a 'register of patients with a diagnosis of cancer excluding non-melanotic skin cancers', diagnosed after 1 April 2003 (6 points).*

It will be possible to search for some cancer patients who are taking long-term drugs such as tamoxifen or GnRH analogues. Similarly, individual doctors and nurses may be able to name some cancer patients who are known to them. Some practices are using the Macmillan Gold Standards Framework for patients with cancer and so a register already exists. Furthermore, many practices have been referring patients through fast-track clinics so that they are seen within two weeks for suspected cancer. These records should be reviewed to find out which patients had cancer diagnosed as a result of this referral and their names placed on the register.

PCOs will wish to find out how many patients have been added to a practice cancer register in the previous 12 months to compare the expected prevalence of new cases with the reported prevalence. If patients with non-melanotic skin cancers have been added to the register an exception code can be applied.

Ongoing management

CANCER 2. Review. *The percentage of patients with cancer diagnosed from 1 April 2003 with a review by the practice, recorded within six months of confirmation of the diagnosis. This should include an assessment of support needs, if any, and a review of co-ordination arrangements with secondary care (6 points). (Minimum threshold = 25%, Maximum threshold = 90%.)*

It is important with all disease conditions that are referred to secondary care that shared care takes place so that patients continue to be followed up in primary care.

Cancer is no exception and in those patients where their cancer is progressive and spreads there will be considerable social, psychological and medical needs. Some patients will be going through recognised psychological reactions such as anger, denial and depression and a review at six months after the diagnosis has been made will be very helpful to these patients. This provides an opportunity to assess a patient's needs and also those of their carer and to co-ordinate care with secondary care as appropriate. There is no reason why these reviews cannot continue if they are clinically indicated and other members of the team are involved as appropriate.

Total points available for Cancer = 12

Mental Health

Mental health problems are common in practice and there will be difficulties in setting up a disease register as a decision needs to be made as to which patients have severe mental illness and those that do not. Mental health conditions that might fulfil these criteria are psychotic illnesses, for example schizophrenia, depression, severe anxiety disorders and many other conditions such as eating disorders. The initiation of such a register is so that these patients may be identified and reviewed on a regular basis, particularly those who are vulnerable members of the community as a result of their mental illness.

Mental Health is also represented in the new contract under the NES for Depression and under the organisational domains, e.g., follow-up of patients receiving depot injections (Medicines Management 7).

There are five separate quality indicators, with the abbreviation MH for Mental Health, with a total of 41 points.

Records

MH 1. Disease register. *The practice can produce a register of people with severe long-term mental health problems who require and have agreed to regular follow-up (7 points).*

For each individual practice, it would be helpful to have a multidisciplinary practice meeting to come to a decision as to which mental illness in individual patients constitutes the category of severe mental health – in addition, to identify individual patients who would be appropriate to include in this category, particularly those with chronic mental health problems such as schizophrenia. Similarly, community psychiatric nurses may also be able to identify patients who are eligible for this register. The great difficulty of this quality indicator is that there is no exact definition of which patients should be included on the register. Patients with long-term depression, particularly those where there is a known risk of suicide, must be included. The register needs to be flexible and regularly updated.

Ongoing Management

MH 2. Review. *The percentage of patients with severe long-term mental health problems with a review recorded in the preceeding 15 months. This review includes a check on the accuracy of prescribed medication, a review of physical health and a review of* *co-ordination arrangements with secondary care (23 points). (Minimum threshold = 25%, Maximum threshold = 90%.)*

There are a considerable number of points available for this quality indicator and having created a register it is important that a recall system is put into place. This may be using prescription review dates as a reminder. At these reviews it is important to consider whether the medication is being prescribed as appropriate, the compliance and whether it should be continued and at what dose. When reviewing physical health it is important to consider factors such as alcohol intake, smoking and other diseases such as heart disease. Similarly it is an opportunity to review the input of other healthcare workers and the role that any secondary care services are providing. In relation to informal carers, this is an opportunity to create a register of such carers which is discussed later in the organisational domain of management.

MH 3. Lithium levels. *The percentage of patients on lithium therapy with a record of lithium levels checked within the previous six months (3 points). (Minimum threshold = 25%, Maximum threshold = 90%.)*

Lithium therapy is used in the treatment of hypomania (sometimes called bipolar depression). Unfortunately, the therapeutic window for lithium is narrow and if it is prescribed in a dose for an individual patient where the serial levels are more than 1mmol/l, then over a prolonged period toxicity may result affecting the kidneys, thyroid gland and nervous system. It is therefore important that patients on lithium have their levels monitored regularly. Most practices are likely to have relatively few patients who are taking lithium and a register of these patients may be made by searching the computer prescribing programme for patients who are taking lithium. It is important that these patients are given reminders for blood tests every quarter.

Practical point
Where these blood tests are being undertaken by secondary care, the results should be requested for individual patients' medical records.

MH 4. Lithium and testing of creatinine and TSH. *The percentage of patients on lithium therapy with a record of serum creatinine and TSH in the preceding 15 months (3 points). (Minimum threshold = 25%, Maximum threshold = 90%.)*

When requesting lithium levels it is important that on an annual basis serum creatinine and TSH (thyroid stimulating hormone) are also requested and again if these blood tests are being undertaken by secondary care services that this information is passed on to the practice. This will have the benefit of improving shared care arrangements between primary and secondary care.

MH 5. Lithium levels in therapeutic range. *The percentage of patients on lithium therapy with a record of lithium levels in the therapeutic range within the previous six months (5 points). (Minimum threshold = 25%, Maximum threshold = 70%.)*

Where patients on lithium levels are not within the therapeutic range, it is important to review their medication and organise for a further blood test at an appropriate interval.

Total points available for Mental Health = 41

Asthma

Asthma is one of the most common chronic diseases in the UK and varies greatly in severity between individuals. As discussed previously some patients labelled with asthma where there is reduced reversibility of their symptoms may actually have COPD. It is believed that up to 8% of the community may suffer with asthma and it is becoming increasingly recognised and more commonly diagnosed in childhood.

Asthma clinics have been run for many years in general practice through the previous GP contract and as a result hospital admissions have stopped increasing and deaths from asthma now appear to be declining. This has been achieved through a regular structured review for patients with asthma undertaken by practice nurses who have received specialist training. Therefore, for many practices the quality indicators that relate to asthma will be an extension of work that is already being undertaken.

There are seven separate quality indicators denoted by ASTHMA with a total of 72 points.

Records

ASTHMA 1. Disease register. *The practice can produce a register of patients with asthma excluding patients with asthma who have been prescribed no asthma-related drugs in the last 12 months (7 points).*

As stated in the introduction, it will hopefully not be too big a test to produce an asthma register and perhaps even more straightforward as it will be possible to exclude those individual patients who have not been prescribed asthma-related medication in the last 12 months.

Initial management

ASTHMA 2. Confirmation of diagnosis. *The percentage of patients age eight and over diagnosed as having asthma from 1 April 2003 where the diagnosis has been confirmed by spirometry or peak flow measurement (15 points). (Minimum threshold = 25%, Maximum threshold = 70%.)*

In order to make the diagnosis of asthma it is important either to have performed spirometry or serial peak flow measurements which demonstrate variability or reversibility with appropriate medication.

Ongoing management

ASTHMA 3. Smoking status age 14 to 19. *The percentage of patients with asthma between the ages of 14 and 19 in whom there is a record of smoking status in the* *previous 15 months (6 points). (Minimum threshold = 25%, Maximum threshold = 70%.)*

As stated for many of the other quality indicators, it is important to enquire about smoking status as appropriate at each consultation and in relation to asthma this needs to be done from the age of 14 years onwards. However, it should be appreciated that this is an exercise to gain points under the new contract as individuals in this age group may not wish to admit that they smoke.

ASTHMA 4. Smoking status age 20 and over. *The percentage of patients age 20 and over with asthma whose notes record smoking status in the past 15 months, except those who have never smoked where smoking status should be recorded at least once (6 points). (Minimum threshold = 25%, Maximum threshold = 70%.)*

This is similar to the last indicator, but applies to patients over the age of 20 years. This information is likely to be more accurate in this group than for the last group for the reasons stated under ASTHMA 3.

ASTHMA 5. Smoking cessation advice. *The percentage of patients with asthma who smoke, and whose notes contain a record that smoking cessation advice has been offered within last 15 months (6 points). (Minimum threshold = 25%, Maximum threshold = 70%.)*

As in all chronic disease conditions smoking cessation advice is important, particularly in young patients as those who smoke are more likely to go on and develop conditions such as COPD.

Practical point

More than 20% of deaths in the UK are related to smoking. There are 87 quality indicator points to be gained in relation to smoking (status and cessation advice) and so almost one-tenth of the QOF distributed through several of the chronic diseases of the clinical domain. It is important that practices develop policies in relation to the recording of smoking status and the delivery of smoking cessation advice. Efforts in this area will not only reduce morbidity and mortality in individual practices, but they will claim reward through quality indicator points.

ASTHMA 6. Asthma review. *The percentage of patients with asthma who have had an asthma review in the last 15 months (20 points). (Minimum threshold = 25%, Maximum threshold = 70%.)*

Asthma is a common problem and so to ensure that all patients on the asthma disease register have had an annual review is a big task which is perhaps made slightly easier as the maximum threshold in this condition is 70%. The 'Blue Book' referred to earlier suggests that an asthma review should first assess symptoms through three questions:

1   Has your asthma affected your sleeping, e.g., through a cough?
2   Have you had your usual asthma symptoms during the day?
3   Has your asthma interfered with your usual activities of daily living?

In addition, an asthma review should include:

- a peak flow measurement to compare with the previous 'best' peak flow reading
- assessment of inhaler technique
- consideration of a personalised asthma plan.

This is also an opportunity to review medication and a peak flow diary. As a result of the enormity of the task some practices are considering a possible review by telephone, particularly for those patients who default from review and so maybe some of those most at risk of complications of asthma.

ASTHMA 7. Influenza vaccination. *The percentage of patients age 16 years and over with asthma who have had influenza immunisation in the preceding 1 September to 31 March (12 points). (Minimum threshold = 25%, Maximum threshold = 70%.)*

For respiratory conditions such as asthma it is important to advocate vaccination where it is not contraindicated as people with asthma who contract infection with influenza may experience increased respiratory distress. In addition, they are more likely to need medication with oral steroids and are more likely to require hospital admission.

Total points available for Asthma = 72

Practical point
Each chronic disease should not necessarily be considered in isolation as they have been in this chapter. Many diseases co-exist, e.g., hypertension, diabetes and CHD. Care should be 'joined up' for such patients so that there are not separate reviews for each chronic disease that they suffer with. This approach, which centres on the person and not the disease, can reduce workload and increase efficiency. This should be taken into account when a recall system is being put into place for each one of the ten chronic diseases of the QOF.

Exception Reporting

For a variety of reasons, some practices may be able to provide a good argument as to why certain patients should not be included in relation to the QOF targets as they may be making the maximum threshold percentage difficult to obtain.

For this reason the quality framework allows certain patients to be excluded or exempt from disease registers or the outcome targets or the process targets for an individual chronic disease. This will be permissible if an individual patient cannot fulfil the defined quality indicator criteria for reasons that are outside the control of the doctor. This forms the basis of what is referred to as 'exception reporting' and there are nine possible exception criteria which may be applied to the ten chronic diseases of the clinical domain of the QOF. These are divided into three areas which are:

1   exclusion from the disease register
2   exclusion from the outcome targets
3   exclusion from the process targets.

The criteria for these three areas of exclusion are as follows.

1 Exclusion from the disease register

- A patient who has defaulted three review invitations in the preceding 12 months.
- A circumstance where chronic disease review may be inappropriate: for example, a patient who is terminally ill.
- For a new patient, or where a patient is newly diagnosed with a chronic disease, the practice has three months' 'grace' before they are included in the disease register.

2 Exclusion from the outcome targets

- A patient who is on maximum doses of appropriate medication: for example, a statin to reduce serum cholesterol but their cholesterol remains greater than 5 mmol/l.
- A patient for whom medication may be contraindicated: for example, a patient who has had an allergic reaction or adverse reaction to a beta blocker on the CHD register.
- A patient who cannot tolerate the medication prescribed: for example, the feelings of tiredness and lethargy that are sometimes attributed to beta blocker therapy.
- A situation where a patient does not wish to have investigation or treatment and so gives 'informed dissent'.
- Situations that arise when treatment may make another supervening condition worse: for example, the use of an ACE inhibitor in CHD where a patient has severe renal impairment.

3 Exclusion from the process targets

- Circumstances arise where the necessary investigation or secondary care service is not available: for example, an ECHO to make the diagnosis of heart failure.

Whatever the reason for exception reporting, details must be fully documented in the individual patient record. In the circumstance of informed dissent, this must be carefully recorded and if appropriate the patient should sign to state that they are not consenting. One of the great strengths in the new contract over the 1990 GP contract is the option to exempt patients from targets where patient care cannot be delivered for reasons beyond the doctor's control. This is good patient-centred practice and empowers patients to take an important role in decision making and to take responsibility for their own health. However, it is vital that practices stick rigidly to the criteria defined above as PCOs are likely to perform regular spot checks on patients who have been excluded from targets.

Some GP computer systems do not presently provide the software for exception reporting and in the meantime doctors are strongly encouraged to keep paper records that can then be entered into the computer system at a later date.

The exception reporting framework allows for exceptions in three possible categories:

- An entire indicator group: for example, the disease register. In terms of calculating the threshold percentage this means that the total number of patients within the disease register is reduced by one.
- A specific single indicator: for example, a single indicator such as cholesterol level. In terms of calculating the threshold percentage this means that the patient will not be excluded from the remaining indicators in that disease category.
- Other exception types: for example, where a particular investigation is not available this means that calculations will need to be adjusted at a local level and so be determined by the local PCO.

Further advice regarding exception reporting and how it will affect points and payments to the practice can be obtained from the local PCO and should be studied carefully.

An example of a quality indicator that may require possible exception reporting is the disputed COPD quality indicator, COPD 3 – spirometry including reversibility testing. In view of the conflict with NICE guidelines, exception reporting may be a possible way of opting out of performing reversibility testing. Again it is important to obtain guidance and agreement as appropriate from the local PCO.

Tips for the clinical domain of the QOF

The ten chronic disease conditions have been discussed in detail. In order to obtain a high proportion of the 550 quality indicator points available in the clinical domain it is important to:

- become familiar with the ten chronic disease conditions and their individual computer templates and the clinical data required. In addition, refer as required to the 'Blue Book' (nGMS Contract) Supporting Documentation
- when entering data on the computer ensure it is Read coded correctly as are any computer templates, otherwise your efforts cannot be rewarded
- when diagnosing one of the ten chronic diseases, enter the confirmatory diagnostic test(s)
- record smoking status where possible and whether smoking cessation advice has been given to smokers
- measure blood pressure opportunistically
- where appropriate recommend influenza vaccination
- if in doubt, find out.

Finally, there are occasions when a review or partial **review by telephone** may be possible and appropriate for the patient who has not got the time to come and see you – for example, a patient with asthma. It is possible to ask about smoking status and provide smoking cessation advice as appropriate. However, it is more difficult to achieve a complete review as outlined in Asthma quality indicator 6.

CHAPTER 7

Quality and Outcomes Framework: the other domains

The last chapter considered in depth just over 50% of the points under the QOF in relation to the clinical domain and the ten chronic diseases that constitute that domain. The remaining 500 points are comprised as follows:

Organisational Domain	Available points
Records and Information	85
Information for Patients (Communication)	8
Education and Training	29
Practice Management	20
Medicines Management	42
Total	**184**

Additional Services Domain	
Cervical Screening	22
Child Health Surveillance	6
Maternity Services	6
Contraceptive Services	2
Total	**36**

Patient Experience and Linked Payments Domain	
Consultation Length	30
Patient Survey	70
Holistic Care	100
Quality Practice	30
Access Bonus	50
Total	**280**
Total points (with clinical domain of 550)	**1050**

Nearly half the payment under the QOF is for these quality indicators and some practices may have been preoccupied with the ten chronic diseases and setting up annual reviews and putting these indicators to one side. The two parts of the QOF should happen simultaneously and in several areas complement each other and these will be described during this chapter.

Organisational Domains

There are a potential 184 points (nearly one-fifth of the total available for the QOF) for the following organisational domains:

- Records and Information about Patients
- Information for Patients (Communication)
- Education and Training
- Practice Management
- Medicines Management.

Organisational criteria are designed to achieve two functions:

1   to list tasks that are required to prove compliance with legislation or good practice
2   to signpost the organisational tasks required to improve a practice.

Records and Information about Patients

Almost half of the available points for these five organisational domains relate to the medical records and if a practice is not using its computer for all patient contacts, then this should start as soon as possible. This applies to all clinical staff including locums. It also means the entries in the medical records must be made for surgery consultations, prescribing, telephone contacts and home visits and any out-of-hours activity. This is detailed in the first indicator, Records 1. The era of scribbled notes on pieces of paper or 'sticky notes' which many of us use regularly is over! Most GP computer systems have internal email to pass on messages and hopefully in this way information will not get mislaid or lost.

Practical point
The secret to success in this domain is the creation of appropriate protocols and this is discussed further in relation to the individual indicators.

In particular, smoking status and blood pressure measurements feature promi-nently in this domain and so overlap with the clinical domain.

It should also be mentioned that there is overlap between the work required for this organisational domain and the time-limited DES, the 'Quality Information Preparation Payment'. This is discussed in Chapter 3 and there are monies avail-able for medical notes summarising. Although it is only available for 2003/04 and 2004/05, it may be worth in the region of £1000 to £5000 for an average practice.

There are 19 separate quality indicators denoted by Records with a total of 85 points.

Records 1. Recording contacts. *Each patient contact with a clinician is recorded in the patient's record, including consultations, visits and telephone advice (1 point).*

To reiterate an earlier comment: the era of scribbled notes on pieces of paper or 'sticky notes' is over.

Records 2. Legible entries. *Entries in the records are legible (1 point).*

Fortunately, the use of a computer overcomes the frequently quoted adage of doctors' bad handwriting, but it is still possible to make typing errors and care should be taken to read entries of free text after they have been typed.

Records 3. Records out of hours. *The practice must have a system for transferring and acting on information about patients seen by other doctors out of hours (1 point).*

This will vary regionally as some out-of-hours services may have a direct computer link, while others may need to transfer the information from other media such as faxes.

Records 4. Messages and visit requests. *There should be a reliable system to ensure that messages and requests for visits are recorded and that the appropriate doctor or team member receives and acts upon them (1 point).*

Like many aspects of the new contract this requires a practice protocol where contact information is acted upon appropriately and audited.

Records 5. Actioning hospital reports and investigations. *The practice should have a system for dealing with any hospital report or investigation results that identifies a responsible health professional and ensures that any necessary action is taken (1 point).*

Like indicator 4 above this will require an agreed practice protocol where fail-safe mechanisms are in place so that any important clinical communications are not overlooked or missed – for example, a patient with a raised glucose. A protocol should define the urgency of particular glucose levels, which clinician is responsible for contacting the patient and how a record can be made that this task has been completed appropriately.

Records 6. Informing team members about the death of a patient. *A system should be in place for ensuring that the relevant team members are informed about patients who have died (1 point).*

Some practices have a discrete whiteboard that can be seen daily by the team for this purpose and a designated member of staff to ensure it is updated as soon as possible and also to enter the details into a permanent death register. Some practices may also enter the date of death in the medical records of a spouse to alert practitioners consulting with this patient in the future.

Records 7. Medication records. *The medicines that a patient is receiving need to be clearly listed in their medical record (1 point).*

Most practices are doing this anyway. However, some practices may need to transfer this information from paper to computer records.

Records 8. Recording of adverse drug reactions. *There is a designated place for the recording of drug allergies and adverse reactions in the notes and these are clearly recorded (1 point).*

Adverse drug reactions including allergies must be flagged up for any clinician who prescribes for a patient. Ideally, this should be computer based when prescribing, but where paper records are used for house visits this information should be clearly written on the front of the notes. Some practices print out a summary of a patient's records for house visits and this summary should also contain adverse drug reactions.

Records 9. Repeat medications. *For repeat medicines, an indication for the drug needs to be identified in the records. This is for drugs added to repeat prescriptions with effect from 1 April 2004. The minimum expected standard for this indicator is 80% (4 points).*

Individual software for GP computer programs needs to be examined as to how this may be achieved.

Records 10. Smoking status of patients. *The smoking status of patients age 15–75 needs to be recorded for at least 55% of patients (6 points).*

The only way of monitoring this is electronically and practices that have regularly entered three-year checks and new patient registration checks under the previous contract may already have achieved the 55% target. If not, then it is important to enter this information at each consultation, and for patients other than those who have been Read coded as having 'never smoked', this information should be appropriately updated. It has considerable relevance to the health of the practice population.

Records 11. Blood pressure measurements. *The blood pressure of patients age 45 and over is recorded in the preceding five years for at least 55% of patients (10 points).*

A computer search will reveal how much work requires to be done by a practice. Recalling patients and opportunistic measurements are likely to create further work as patients with borderline readings or high readings are detected and need to be reviewed. However, this is good clinical practice and also relevant to several of the indicators of the clinical domain.

Records 12. *When a member of the team prescribes a medicine other than a non-medicated dressing, topical treatment or over-the-counter (OTC) medicine there is a mechanism for that prescription to be entered into the patient's general practice record (2 points).*

This is particularly important in the case of nurse and midwife prescribing. It may be that not all GP practice computer systems will have the software to perform this task so free text entry on the computer may be necessary. A method of auditing this process needs to be put in place. It is important also that all doctors prescribe using the computer and not by hand.

Records 13. Dying patients and the out-of-hours service. *There is a system to alert the out-of-hours service or duty doctor to patients dying at home (2 points).*

Some practices will be opting out of hours including Saturday mornings and so with further use of out-of-hours services this will be an increasing issue for many practices. Professionals caring for dying patients out of hours need to have adequate details in relation to their diagnosis, medication and carers. For example, faxing these details on a regular basis to the out-of-hours service is one method and the information should be updated as each patient's clinical condition changes or deteriorates. Out-of-hours services generally use computers and this information may then be inputted onto their computer systems. This is good practice to optimise patient care should a problem arise out of hours with a dying patient and ensure continuity of care, particularly if a 'crisis' situation arises.

Records 14. Filing of patient records. *The records, hospital letters and investigation reports are filed in date order or available electronically in date order (3 points).*

This may already apply to many written records and is easiest to do with A4 records. For paperless practices the task may be easier still, but long periods of time may be spent scanning letters. For those practices with electronic laboratory links the information will automatically be entered in patients' records. However, it should be remembered that the creation of electronic records or increased use of such records does not render everything in a manual record immediately redundant.

Records 15. Record summaries. *The practice has up-to-date clinical summaries in at least 60% of patient records (25 points).*

The ideal way to do this is on the computer system and this will have benefits for the clinical and organisational domains. For example, it will help with the establishment of disease registers. For many practices this is likely to be a huge task and it may be necessary to employ appropriate individuals to help with summarising. A protocol should be drawn up not just in relation to performing the summaries and what information is significant, but how patient records will be updated in the future and the summary of new patients and their records when they arrive at the practice. It also has benefits for practices wishing to teach undergraduates or be training practices for postgraduates, e.g., GP registrars. This indicator is worth 25 points, but potentially much more than these as described.

Records 16. Smoking status. *The smoking status of patients age 15–75 is recorded for at least 75% of patients (5 points).*

This is an extension of the indicator Records 10 and will require regular computer entries as detailed in the indicator Records 10.

Records 17. Blood pressure measurements. *The blood pressure of patients age 45 and over is recorded in the preceding five years for at least 75% of patients (5 points).*

This is an extension of the indicator Records 11 and will require regular computer entries as detailed in the indicator Records 11.

Records 18. Record summaries. *The practice has up-to-date clinical summaries in at least 80% of patient records (8 points).*

This is an extension of the indicator Records 15 and will require regular computer entries as detailed in the indicator Records 15.

Records 19. New patients and record summaries. *80% of newly registered patients have had their notes summarised within eight weeks of receipt of their medical records by the practice (7 points).*

Ideally, these notes should be summarised as soon as they arrive and the dates the notes arrived should be recorded and when they are summarised to enable audit of this indicator. This should also be taken care of through an adequate practice protocol which also includes a method to achieve indicator 15 as described above.

Total points available for Records = 85

Information for Patients (Communication)

This is a relatively small part of the organisational domain of the new contract where there are eight separate quality indicators denoted by Information with a total of 8 points. All refer to information that should be available to patients and particularly the role of the telephone relating to access.

Information 1. Telephone access to out-of-hours service. *The practice has a system to allow patients to contact the out-of-hours service by making no more than two telephone calls (0.5 point).*

This is likely to require an answering system which provides the number of the out-of-hours provider for the patient to call and an agreement with the out-of-hours provider that no further telephone call will be required. This system should be tested each working day.

Information 2. Answerphone messages. *If an answering system is used out of hours, the message should be clear and the contact number should be given at least twice (0.5 point).*

The answering system should be tested each working day and ensure no unwanted background noise and where tapes are used they should be renewed as appropriate.

Information 3. Telephone access during the day. *The practice has arrangements for patients to speak to GPs and nurses on the telephone during the working day (1 point).*

These calls should be logged and carefully detailed in the medical records. If you are calling a patient back because you were busy and there is no reply, this should also be recorded.

Information 4. Removing patients from the list. *If a patient is removed from a practice's list, the practice should carefully provide an explanation of the reasons in writing to the patient and information on how to find a new practice, unless it is perceived such an action would result in a violent response by the patient (1 point).*

In addition, it is important to record what attempts have been made to prevent and redeem the breakdown of doctor–patient relationships in each individual case.

Information 5. Smoking cessation. *The practice should support smokers in stopping by a strategy, which includes providing literature and offering appropriate therapy (2 points).*

It is important to draw up a practice protocol with use of posters in the waiting room and easy access to relevant patient information leaflets. Details regarding smoking cessation consultations should be available and the medications that are available through the practice such as nicotine replacement therapy (NRT) and bupropion.

Information 6. Information on antenatal and postnatal care. *Information should be available to patients on the roles of the GP, community midwife, health visitor and hospital clinics in the provision of antenatal and postnatal care (0.5 point).*

Ideally, this could be an information pack together with the contact details for any of the relevant healthcare professionals.

Information 7. Access to receptionist. *Patients should be able to access a receptionist via the telephone or face to face in the practice, for at least 45 hours over 5 days, Monday to Friday except where agreed with the PCO (1.5 points).*

This means availability of contact on average nine hours per day. The exact spread of this contact can be negotiated with the local PCO and where direct access may not be possible, it is vital that urgent calls can be directed appropriately and when direct access will resume.

Information 8. Accessing the out-of-hours service by telephone. *The practice has a system to allow patients to contact the out-of-hours service by making no more than one telephone call (1 point).*

Telephone systems are available that will do this, but they can be expensive. Some practices may already achieve this as their calls are diverted through NHS Direct.

The practice leaflet

It might be thought that this organisational domain would reward practices for providing a quality practice leaflet. Unfortunately, this is not the case and these have to be revised by 1 August 2004 in line with paragraph 75 of Schedule 6 and Schedule 10 of the GMS Contracts Regulations 2004.

The information to be included in practice leaflets is detailed in Schedule 3 of the GMS contract.

Total points available for Information for Patients = 8

Education and Training

Many practices may already be conducting this activity. If not, then the writing of the relevant practice policies electronically means that they will be available for all staff. In addition, it is important that the practice manager keeps files of activity in this organisational domain as evidence to the PCO to claim the available points.

There are nine separate quality indicators denoted by Education with a total of 29 points.

Education 1. Basic life-support skills training for clinical staff. *There is a record of all practice-employed clinical staff having attended training/updating in basic life-support skills in the preceding 18 months (4 points).*

At first glance this might seem easy to achieve, but imagine a large practice where there are new members of staff and some members of staff missed the training session as they were on leave. Evidence of training (certificates) should be kept carefully by the practice manager as well as copies kept in individual personal staff portfolios.

Education 2. Significant event reviews. *The practice has undertaken a minimum of six significant event reviews in the past three years (4 points).*

It is useful to keep a log of significant events and then a reflection of each entry together with learning points. This requires both organised significant event review meetings and careful recording of the minutes of these meetings. As this indicator refers to 'the practice' it is expected that such reviews involve several members of the team and therefore that they are multidisciplinary. A file should be created for these meetings as evidence that they have taken place. It should also be stated that significant events are not necessarily critical incidents, but they can be events regarding good practice. This information will also be important for inclusion in GP appraisal and revalidation folders.

Education 3. Nurse appraisal. *All practice-employed nurses have an annual appraisal (2 points).*

This should follow national guidelines and ensure clinical input. This can lead into indicator 8 below as the appraisal should result in the identification of learning needs and so the writing of a personal learning plan. This can be reviewed at annual appraisal. Again a file should be created for these meetings as evidence that they have taken place, together with the paperwork.

Education 4. Induction training. *All new staff receive induction training (3 points).*

It may be helpful to create an induction information pack that can be used for all new staff and those in training, e.g., GP registrars, who are changing posts regularly.

Education 5. Basic life-support skills training for all staff. *There is a record of all practice-employed staff having attended training/updating in basic life-support skills in the preceding 36 months (3 points).*

The fact that this refers to all staff means that if one member of staff has not had approved training, the practice will not be eligible for these points. However, one assumes that the PCO would allow a proportion of these points to be claimed in such a scenario.

Education 6. Patient complaints. *The practice conducts an annual review of patient complaints and suggestions to ascertain general learning points that are shared with the team (3 points).*

Most practices will have a complaints system in place, but perhaps as part of practice meetings these should be shared with team and be learning opportunities. Again these should be carefully recorded as the PCO will expect minutes to be available as evidence of attainment of this and other indicators.

Education 7. Significant event reviews. *The practice has undertaken a minimum of 12 significant event reviews in the past three years which include (if these have occurred) (4 points):*

- *any death occurring on the practice premises*
- *two new cancer diagnoses*
- *two deaths where terminal care has taken place at home*
- *one patient complaint*
- *one suicide*
- *one section under the Mental Health Act.*

In order to gain all 4 points, this assumes that practices will have held such reviews prior to the start of the new contract. Otherwise this would mean conducting monthly reviews. It may be possible to combine this with the Education 6 indicator above. In relation to significant event reviews where there are critical incidents it will be helpful to consider what happened and why, if the persons involved were aware and has it been a learning experience for the team where change can be demonstrated to prevent a similar incident in the future.

Education 8. Nurse personal learning plans. *All practice-employed nurses have personal learning plans which have been reviewed at annual appraisal (3 points).*

As stated earlier (Education 3) this should be a routine part of appraisal.

Education 9. Appraisal of non-clinical team members. *All practice-employed non-clinical team members have an annual appraisal (3 points).*

Although there is no stated requirement for them to write personal learning plans, it would be good practice and helpful to enable team development and incorporated into the practice professional development plan (PPDP).

Total points available for Education = 29

Practice Management

A relatively small number of points are available for this organisational domain when one bears in mind the multiple roles or multitasking of a practice manager. These include being reactive as an administrator and a manager, but also being proactive as a strategic planner. Even though the new contract has been carefully defined in relation to targets, planning and organisation is required to meet the targets for an individual practice.

Key roles for practice managers include workable practice policies, e.g., in relation to instrument sterilisation – similarly, the agreement and adherence to protocols which may be those of the practice or local and national protocols. Patient and staff safety is also a huge task and perhaps not given due reward in this domain. Similarly, the role of the practice manager is not adequately reflected through the awarding of points in this domain, but various aspects of a practice manager's roles appear in the other domains.

There are ten separate quality indicators denoted by Management with a total of 20 points.

Management 1. Child protection. *Individual healthcare professionals have access to information on local procedures relating to child protection (1 point).*

It is important that the practice has a copy of the local child protection procedures and that it can be accessed on the practice intranet or through the practice manager. All relevant staff must know how to access this document and have seen and read it and perhaps discussed important points from the document in a practice meeting. This information should be minuted as evidence for meeting the criteria to claim this indicator point. It may also help to arrange a meeting between local child protection experts and the practice team so that they are aware of local procedures and local training courses.

Management 2. Back-up for computer data. *There should be clearly defined arrangements for backing up computer data, back-up verification, safe storage of back-up tapes and authorisation for loading programs where a computer is used (1.5 points).*

The policy for this needs to be clearly defined by the practice manager and who is responsible for carrying out these tasks and who will deputise for them when the manager or other designated staff member is on leave. This policy may include the storing of weekly back-up tapes in a fire-proof safe or off site taking care to adhere to confidentiality issues – in addition, the replacement of back-up tapes at regular intervals.

Management 3. Hepatitis B status of clinical staff. *The hepatitis B status of all doctors and relevant practice employed staff is to be recorded and immunisation recommended if required in accordance with national guidance (0.5 point).*

This is important for the safety of staff and this information together with relevant laboratory reports should be kept by the practice manager confidentially. For staff who are not immunised, a vaccination course should be offered after the hepatitis B surface antigen level has been assayed and their antibody response tested two months after the course. Similarly, staff who are immune should be re-tested perhaps every three to five years to ensure that they continue to be immune and whether or not a booster vaccination is required. If the practice manager is made responsible for this an appropriate system of recall can be instituted.

Practical point
Under the Health and Safety Act, practices need to ensure that all staff have had relevant training and have been informed about the health and safety procedures at the practice to ensure a safe working environment.

Management 4. Instrument sterilisation. *The arrangements for instrument sterilisation should comply with national guidelines as applicable to primary care (1 point).*

This should concur with current guidelines from the PCO. Again a practice protocol must be available and its implementation supervised by the practice manager. Following concerns regarding transmission of vCJD (new variant Creutzfeldt-Jakob Disease) some practices now use disposable surgical instruments and vaginal speculums.

Management 5. Appointment system. *The practice should offer a range of appointment times to patients which as a minimum should include morning and afternoon appointments five mornings and four afternoons per week except where agreed with the PCO (3 points).*

There will be overlap with this quality indicator and the access target indictor which is to be discussed later. Where it is not possible to implement this indicator and there are good reasons why it cannot be implemented this should be discussed and negotiated with the local PCO. Information regarding this could be publicised in the practice leaflet.

Management 6. Advertising vacancies. *Person specifications and job descriptions should be produced for all advertised vacancies (2 points).*

The easiest way to start with this indicator is to make sure that up-to-date job descriptions are available for all currently employed staff. Similarly, as employment law changes these descriptions should be updated so that if a person leaves their post, their vacancy is advertised, which is current with new employment law legislation. In relation to these job descriptions the practice manager should update potential job descriptions taking into account circulars from the Equal Opportunities Commission, the Disability Discrimination Act, the Commission for Racial Equality and ACAS (the Advisory, Conciliation and Arbitration Service).

Management 7. Practice equipment. *The practice needs to have systems in place to ensure regular and appropriate inspection, calibration, maintenance and replacement of equipment including (3 points):*

- a defined responsible person
- clear recording

- systematic pre-planned schedules
- reporting of faults.

A lot of work is involved with this indicator as this covers equipment from printers, fridges, sphygmomanometers to sterilisers. This may require outside contractors to maintain and calibrate instruments and this can be expensive and require a lot of organisation. Further details may be obtained from the Health and Safety Executive website: www.hse.gov.uk/healthservices/index.htm.

Practical point

A log of inspection and maintenance should be available to see by the PCO if required. All of these form part of the statutory risk assessment undertaken by practices to comply with the 1999 Health and Safety at Work Regulations.

Management 8. Prevention of fraud. *The practice needs to have a policy to ensure the prevention of fraud and have defined levels of financial responsibility and accountability for staff undertaking financial transactions (accounts, payroll, drawings, payment of invoices, signing cheques, petty cash, pensions and superannuation) (1 point).*

Practical point

In relation to the new contract any claim for points under the QOF or for running a Directed Enhanced Service must have a record of the clinical evidence/data to support that claim.

A practical policy should be written and agreed with all business partners and the practice manager and shown to the practice accountant for their feedback. A GP practice involves both running a primary care health service and a business and it makes sound financial sense to be sure mistakes are not made and that fraud does not occur intentionally or unintentionally by anyone working at the practice.

Practical point

Petty cash should be carefully managed with written evidence for income and outgoings. Similarly there should be two signatures on each cheque. To protect individuals from accusations it is important that the same individual in the practice does not place orders, sort out the invoices, sign the cheques and put income into the business account.

Management 9. Informal carers. *The practice should have a protocol for the identification of carers and a mechanism for the referral of carers for social services assessment (3 points).*

Informal carers, e.g. spouses of patients with chronic and severe health needs such as advanced cancer, multiple sclerosis, strokes and deteriorating health as a result of age, provide care 24 hours a day, 365 days a week. They need support and a register should be created to identify these people and ensure that their physical, psychological, social and financial needs are met. One person should be made responsible for regularly updating this register and making sure the needs of informal carers are met where possible – for example, enabling respite care or advising application for an attendance allowance or contact with social services. Relevant information leaflets may also be of help.

Management 10. Staff employment policies. *A written procedure manual should include staff employment policies including equal opportunities, bullying and harassment and sickness absence (including illegal drugs, alcohol and stress) to which staff have access (4 points).*

This follows on from Management indicator number 6. The practice manager should take responsibility for putting this manual together and updating it regularly as legislation changes and inform all staff where the manual is kept and ensure that it is easily accessible. This manual is likely to be inspected during any practice assessment visit.

There is a huge potential workload to meet this Management organisational domain and the ideal person to take overall charge is the practice manager who will need to ensure practice policies are put into place and that individual folders (manual or electronic) are kept for many of the indicators that have been discussed.

Total points available for Management = 20

Medicines Management

Efficient management of medicines should be beneficial to both patients and clinicians alike and should mean that NHS resources are used appropriately. Regular review of repeat prescribing which is a key part of this organisational domain is good practice and similarly the review of emergency medications is very important. Further advice and keeping up to date can be gained by meeting with the PCO prescribing adviser. Any proposed changes should have patient needs at the centre of the changes.

If a practice does not have a robust repeat prescribing policy and system in place then one should be written and agreed with all team members. A practice-based pharmacist can be an invaluable member of the multidisciplinary team for many reasons and also to help implement this organisational domain. It should also be remembered that nearly 25% of the general practice claims settled by the Medical Defence Union are as a result of prescription errors.

There are ten separate quality indicators denoted by the abbreviation Med with a total of 42 points.

Med 1. Record of prescribed medications. *Details of prescribed medicines are available to the prescriber at each surgery consultation (2 points).*

If a practice is using a computer system for all prescribing then the criteria for this quality indicator will have been met. Practices still using a paper-based system and handwritten prescriptions will need to change to using a computer-based system.

Med 2. Anaphylaxis. *The practice should possess the equipment and up-to-date emergency drugs to treat anaphylaxis (2 points).*

There should be a practice policy to check the equipment and to ensure that drugs, such as adrenaline, are in date. It will help to have a written list of medications available on display.

Med 3. Emergency drugs expiry dates. *A system needs to be in place for checking expiry dates of emergency drugs at least on an annual basis (2 points).*

Ideally, this could be a practice pharmacist or another designated individual to perform this and it is probably better performed six monthly rather than annually. The practice policy should be to check drugs on the premises, e.g., in the treatment room and in each doctor's emergency bag, and to replace drugs that have gone past their sell-by date or are about to go past their sell-by date. In relation to the latter, it may be helpful to keep a register of when drugs are due to go out of date.

Med 4. Repeat prescription requests. *The number of hours from requesting a prescription to availability for collection by the patient is 72 hours or less (excluding weekends and bank/local holidays) (3 points).*

It will help to advertise the repeat prescribing system for the practice in the waiting room, in the practice leaflet and on repeat prescriptions. A practice policy on how to achieve this target will help, particularly when doctors are on leave or bank holidays are approaching, such as Christmas and New Year.

Med 5. Medication reviews. *A medication review is recorded in the notes in the preceding 15 months for all patients being prescribed four or more repeat medicines (excluding OTC and topical medications): Standard 80% (7 points).*

Again this quality indicator will require the use of a computer-based repeat prescribing system where annual review dates can be set. These reviews can be planned or performed opportunistically and the review Read coded once it has been performed and it can be undertaken by a GP, nurse or the practice-based pharmacist. The practice will require a clearly defined policy on repeat prescribing. Where a computer program has been set which details the number of repeat prescriptions for a particular medication before a patient is reviewed, this should not be ignored and overridden.

Med 6. Meeting PCO prescribing adviser. *The practice should meet with the PCO prescribing adviser at least annually and agree up to three actions related to prescribing (4 points).*

It is important that the practice appoints a person to lead on prescribing who can attend these meetings, review the Prescribing Analysis and Cost (PACT) data and local PCO prescribing initiatives and disseminate the three actions to the rest of the team.

Med 7. Injectable neuroleptic medication. *Where the practice has responsibility for administering regular injectable neuroleptic medication, there is a system to identify and follow up patients who do not attend (4 points).*

This medication may be administered in the practice or by a member of the local community mental health team. In both scenarios this needs to be recorded and as it may involve a relatively small number of patients, a practice may decide to do this manually. This register could be kept with the neuroleptic medication.

Med 8. Repeat prescription requests. *The number of hours from requesting a prescription to availability for collection by the patient is 48 hours or less (excluding weekends and bank/local holidays) (6 points).*

This is an extension of the Med 4 indicator above, but should still be a target that many practices can meet. For the purposes of audit it will help to enter the date of request of a repeat prescription and when it has been issued. It may be more difficult to enter the date that it has been signed by a doctor.

Med 9. Repeat medication reviews. *A medication review is recorded in the notes in the preceding 15 months for all patients being prescribed repeat medicines (excluding OTC and topical medications): Standard 80% (8 points).*

This is a further extension of the Med 5 indicator above and will require a lot of work.

Med 10. Repeat prescription requests and evidence of change. *The practice meets with the PCO prescribing advisor at least annually, has agreed up to three actions related to prescribing and has subsequently provided evidence of change (4 points).*

The prescribing lead in the practice must ensure that all practice staff are aware of the agreed changes (three actions) and devise a way of searching the computer to provide evidence that these changes have occurred following an audit.

Total points available for Medicines Management = 42

Additional Services Domain

The third quality domain comprises the following additional services:

- Cervical Screening
- Child Health Surveillance
- Maternity Services
- Contraceptive Services.

There are 36 quality indicator points available for this domain and so a relatively small proportion of the total available 1050 points for the QOF. They are all areas which were covered by the previous 1990 GP contract and areas of health promotion in relation to women's health and child health.

Cervical Screening (CS)

There are six separate quality indicators for Cervical Screening denoted by the abbreviation CS with a total of 22 points.

CS 1. Recording of cervical smears. *The percentage of patients aged 25 to 64 years (in Scotland 25–60 years) whose notes record that a cervical smear has been performed in the last three to five years (Standard: 25 to 80%) (11 points)*

This is similar to the targets of the previous 1990 GP contract. However, there is not a lower and a higher target, but rather a gradation. Exception reporting is available for women who have had hysterectomies that involve complete removal of the cervix. Furthermore, following the wording of this indicator means that a cervical smear needs to have been performed, but does not necessarily need to be negative. This latter issue is covered by indicator CS 2 below.

CS 2. Follow-up of inadequate/abnormal smears. *The practice has a system to ensure inadequate/abnormal smears are followed up (3 points).*

Most practices will already have this in place as a result of meeting cytology targets under the 1990 GP contract.

CS 3. Cervical smear defaulters. *The practice has a policy on how to identify and follow up cervical smear defaulters. Patients may opt for exclusion from the cervical cytology recall register by completing a written statement which is filed in the patient record (exception reporting) (2 points).*

As for CS 2 above, most practices will already have this in place as a result of meeting cytology targets under the 1990 GP contract. However, exception reporting for informed dissent was not possible under the 1990 GP contract and is a considerable advance taking into account patient autonomy.

CS 4. Five-yearly recall on exclusions. *Women who have opted for exclusion from the cervical cytology recall register must be offered the opportunity to change their decision at least every five years (2 points).*

Women who have opted out must be provided with the opportunity every five years to reconsider their decision if they wish through an appropriate reminder letter. A system must be in place to identify and recall these women and the person whose responsibility it is to run this system.

CS 5. Cervical smear results. *The practice has a system for informing all women of the results of cervical smears (2 points).*

This can be done by a letter from the practice or an NHS service provider outside of the practice. When the PCO visits the practice for assessment purposes a copy of this letter should be available to view.

CS 6. Audit of cervical screening service. *The practice has a policy for auditing its cervical screening service, and performs an audit of inadequate cervical smears in relation to individual smear takers at least every two years (2 points).*

Audit is important in clinical practice to ascertain if service standards are being met. Furthermore, this audit will enable the practice to look at the performance of smear takers which could be compared to the cytology laboratory's average for inadequate smears.

Total points available for Cervical Screening = 22

Child Health Surveillance (CHS)

There is one separate quality indicator for Child Health Surveillance denoted by the abbreviation CHS with a total of 6 points.

CHS 1. Child development checks. *Child development checks are offered at the intervals agreed in local guidelines and problems are followed up (6 points).*

A system for Child Health Surveillance should be in place at the practice that follows local or national guidelines. The practice should be able to demonstrate that any problems identified are being followed up.

Total points available for Child Health Surveillance = 6

Maternity Services (MAT)

There is one separate quality indicator for Maternity Services denoted by the abbreviation MAT with a total of 6 points.

MAT 1. Antenatal care and screening. *Antenatal care and screening are offered according to current local guidelines (6 points).*

Maternity services should follow local guidelines in relation to antenatal care and screening and be able to demonstrate this by illustration with a case report.

Total points available for Maternity Services = 6

Contraceptive Services (CON)

There are two separate quality indicators for Contraceptive Services denoted by the abbreviation CON with a total of 2 points.

CON 1. Emergency contraception. *The team has a written policy for responding to requests for emergency contraception (1 point).*

This affects the whole practice team including receptionists and the awareness of how to handle requests for emergency contraception with emergency contraception time constraints. Emergency contraception is the term used for preventing conception after intercourse where there has been no contraception used or where it is thought that the contraception used may not have been adequate or effective. Two types of emergency contraception are currently available:

1 'the morning after pill' – which should be taken within 72 hours of unprotected sex, but is most effective if taken in the first 24 hours

2   insertion of a copper IUCD up to five days after presumed ovulation can be used
     for emergency postcoital contraception.

CON 2. Preconception advice. *The team has a policy for providing preconceptual advice*
(1 point).

A practice policy should be available to all practitioners in the practice who may
need to give preconception advice and this should cover areas such as:

- smoking
- alcohol
- substance abuse
- diet
- prophylactic folic acid
- rubella antibody status
- genetically inherited conditions
- pre-existing medical conditions, e.g., diabetes.

Total points available for Contraceptive Services = 2

Patient Experience Domain

The fourth quality domain is Patient Experience for which there are 100 points and
so nearly one-tenth of the total payment for the QOF. This relates to two issues:

- the length of consultations
- patient satisfaction surveys.

This is an area of the contract that encourages practices to be further patient-
centred.

Patient Experience

There are four separate quality indicators for Patient Experience denoted by the
abbreviation PE with a total of 100 points and so almost 10% of the available
points for the QOF.

PE 1. Duration of patient appointments. *The length of routine booked appointments*
with the doctors in the practice is not less than ten minutes. [If the practice routinely sees
extras during booked surgeries, then the average booked consultation length should allow
for the average number of extras seen in a surgery session. If the extras are seen at the
end, then it is not necessary to make this adjustment.]
    For practices with only an open surgery system, the average face-to-face time spent by
the GP with the patient is at least eight minutes.
    For practices that routinely operate a mixed economy of booked and open surgeries they
should report on both criteria.

A total of 30 points are available for this quality indicator.
    Even for those practices who routinely offer ten-minute appointments this is not
an easy target to achieve as extras should not be 'slotted in' during routine booked
appointments unless it can be demonstrated that this does not reduce the duration

of booked appointments. They should therefore be seen at the end of booked appointments. Overall, 75% or more of all appointments should be booked at ten-minute intervals or longer.

Practical point
What happens on a particularly busy day or when a partner is ill or on leave?
Practices will need to demonstrate what their usual practice is by timing the actual length of all consultations over two sample weeks each year.

There are two ways to audit this for inspection by the PCO: first, to have a hand-written appointments book where all appointments are written at ten-minute inter-vals; second, to use the appointments program or your GP computer system. This will record the time a consultation was booked for, when it started and when it finished. It can be seen that there are advantages to both systems in terms of audit. One person needs to take responsibility to oversee this system such as a senior receptionist or the practice manager.

For those practices that run open surgeries the criteria are different as stated above. For practices that run a mixed system, further guidance is available in the 'Blue Book' previously referred to.

PE 2. Approved annual patient survey. *The practice will have to undertake an approved patient survey each year (40 points).*

This must be an approved survey in the preceding year of which there are two.

1   The General Practice Assessment Questionnaire (GPAQ) which can be found on the website: www.gpaq.info.

This has been produced by the University of Manchester and has two versions – one to be used following a visit to the doctor at the practice and the other which is a version to be sent by post. There is no fee for the use of this questionnaire for 'practices who carry out their own surveys' but it is requested that you send a copy of your GPAQ data to the National Primary Care Research and Development Centre at the University of Manchester as detailed on the website so that the data can be added anonymously to national bench-marks.

Or

2   The Improving Practice Questionnaire (IPQ) which may be found on the following website: www.cfep.net.

This questionnaire is copyright and there is a fee for its use. However, this comes with a full analysis and feedback service. The website gives full details of how to make contact with the Client-Focused Evaluations Programme which is based at the University of Exeter.

At present these are the only approved questionnaires to use with this quality domain of the new contract. It is recommended that the reader consult their local PCO to check that they also approve the use of these questionnaires or whether there is one in the locality that they would prefer to be used.

The practice must receive 25 questionnaires per 1000 patients (approximately 50 questionnaires per doctor). These can be administered in two ways. First, on consecutive patients after they have seen the doctor at the surgery, which is thought to reduce bias, or by post, distributed at random. The former is probably easier as responses to postal surveys are often generally poor.

PE 3. Reflection on an approved patient survey and proposed changes. *The practice will have undertaken a patient survey each year, have reflected on the results and have proposed changes if appropriate (15 points).*

If the practice has gone to the trouble of administering the questionnaire, it would seem to be a good use of resources to analyse and summarise the responses. Changes can then be proposed if these are 'appropriate'.

This information is very useful for GP appraisal and revalidation and so is time well spent for several reasons including the fact that patients will benefit and the practice will be paid for it.

PE 4. Discussion of the patient survey with practice team, PCO and evidence of change. *The practice will have undertaken a patient survey each year and discussed the results as a team and with either a patient group or non-executive director of the PCO. Appropriate changes will have been proposed with some evidence that the changes have been enacted (15 points).*

If the results are discussed with the practice team at a practice meeting various proposals for change can be considered and so the creation of an agenda for when delegated practice members meet to discuss these further with:

● the local Patient-Participation Group (PPG)

or

● a non-executive director of the PCO.

Plans for change can then be implemented, together with the collection of evidence that these changes are taking place. The success or otherwise of these changes can be monitored at the next annual patient survey and hopefully will be able to demonstrate that change has occurred.

This is an activity that will need to be co-ordinated by the practice manager, but will require input from the whole team for it to be successful.

Total points available for Patient Experience = 100

Linked Payments Domain

This is part of the fourth quality domain and comprises 180 quality points as follows:

● Holistic Care – 100
● Quality Practice – 30
● Access Bonus – 50

Holistic Care

Holistic Care amounts to 100 points and although it might appear a small section in this chapter it amounts to nearly 10% of the available points for the QOF.

Practical point
It should be noted that both Holistic Care and Quality Practice indicator points are based on achievement in the clinical and organisational domains respectively.

Holistic Care points are based on the proportion of points scored for the third lowest in the ten clinical domains. There are a possible 100 points. Take the example of the Epilepsy clinical domain where there are a total of 16 points available to claim. If Epilepsy is the third lowest of a practice's ten clinical domains and they had gained 4 points in this domain, then the practice would be awarded $4/16 \times 100 = 25$ points.

Practical point
It is important therefore to achieve as many points as possible in each of the ten clinical domains to score a high number of holistic care points.

Total points available for Holistic Care = 100

Quality Practice

Quality Practice points are based on the proportion of points scored for the third lowest in the five organisational domains. There are a possible 30 points.

Take the example of the Information for Patients organisational domain where there are a total of 8 points available to claim. If Information for Patients is the third lowest of a practice's five organisational domains and they had gained 2 points in this domain, then the practice would be awarded $2/8 \times 30 = 7.5$ points.

Total points available for Quality Practice = 30

Access Bonus

This is for practices that deliver access for patients to:

- a GP (not a named GP) within 48 hours (two working days not including Saturday, Sunday, bank holidays and designated staff training through defined protected learning time initiatives)

and

- a primary care professional (a member of the practice or wider team) within 24 hours (by the end of the following working day not including Saturday,

Sunday, bank holidays and designated staff training through defined protected learning time initiatives).

This will be in line with the Planning and Priorities Framework (PPF) 2003/06 target which reflects the commitments in the NHS Plan for Access. There are 50 points available for this referred to as Access Bonus points.

There is a different definition and so criteria in each of the four countries of the UK. In England it will be similar to the access standards expressed in the National Plan. If a practice achieves the access target as defined in its nation then it is entitled to the 50 Access Bonus points.

For this linked payment, there is no direct link to the four domains of the QOF, but rather the DES of Improved Access.

Total points available for the Access Bonus = 50

Review of the QOF of the new contract

Inevitably, the QOF will need to be reviewed as national guidelines such as those from NICE change as a result of research and a new evidence base. It has already been suggested that some changes are required in relation to some of the COPD quality indicators. The GPC of the BMA has said that it is unlikely that there will be any major revisions until April 2006. The likelihood of any change at the moment is where a quality indicator is demonstrated to be dangerous or unsafe and so in this scenario the QOF would need to be reviewed to take into account the associated sudden change in evidence base.

In addition to evidence base, other issues that would lead to review are as follows:

- advances in healthcare
- changes in legislation
- need for clarification of individual quality indicators
- identification of new areas for quality indicators.

The present framework has been based on the best available research evidence: for example, in relation to hypertension where evidence has been derived from the British Hypertension Society (BHS), NICE and SIGN guidelines. Some inconsistencies have been found with, e.g., NICE guidelines which uses a < 80% predicted cut-off for an FEV1 and the diagnosis of COPD whereas that for the new contract is given a level of < 70% predicted. However, these inconsistencies seem to be relatively few in number.

Perhaps there is one reassurance that can be given to those working in primary care who have been experiencing 'change fatigue' and that is that there is now an opportunity for consolidation of the recent changes as a result of the new contract until April 2006. Inevitably, the QOF cannot remain static and we should look towards 2006 for possible changes following review.

Practice audit and review/assessment

Practices should be prepared for a quality framework visit between October 2004 and January 2005 by the local PCO and each practice should have a QOF lead practitioner. GPs will be required to submit the necessary data/report one month in advance. This will need to cover all the areas for which the contractor (the practice) intends to submit a QOF achievement claim, including details on exception reporting. The required information is set out in the DoH publication, *New GMS Contract 2003: Supplementary Documents*. Further details can also be obtained from the Department of Health website: www.dh.gov.uk.

The assessment team

This is likely to take half a day and an assessment team will probably consist of at least three visitors:

- one of whom should be a GP although this may pose difficulties recruiting enough GPs to undertake this task (this person can however be another health-care professional by agreement between the practice and PCO)
- one assessor will normally be a lay person
- a representative from the PCO.

The visit may also involve the LMC. Members of the assessment team should be selected on the basis of:

- meeting certain competencies
- having received appropriate national training

Considerable preparation will be required by the practice for this visit. The computer programme, QMAS (Quality Management and Analysis System), can be used to show how well a practice is performing under the QOF and it is important to be conversant with this as it is a way of further checking that the work on the QOF is being properly recorded for the practice and the local PCO. In addition, some practices (approximately 5%) will be chosen at random for spot checks to curb potential fraud. In a sense, this is not a new phenomenon as this also occurred in the preceding 1990 GP contract.

Outcomes of the visit

Outcomes of the assessment visit are likely to be as follows:

- an assessment of the practice's likely achievement against the QOF
- a written report
- any recommendations for change, e.g., use of Read codes
- suggested changes required by the practice within one month.

Teamwork and the QOF

It has been said that in business teamwork is one of the most popular buzzwords and a question all GPs need to ask in light of the new contract where the emphasis is on practices rather than individuals is 'Are you a team player?'

Drexel University, Philadelphia, USA, has produced a useful definition of teamwork: 'Teamwork is more than group work. It is an organised process that requires concentration on people as well as the product.'

It is suggested that keys to achieving a successful team whether at a university or a GP practice are:

- members of the team work at establishing an effective team
- members need to accept roles, but appreciate that roles may change
- teamwork requires regular structured meetings
- all team members should keep a record of their activities as part of a portfolio or work diary
- appreciating and valuing that each member of the team has a unique role, different skills and a contribution to make
- where individuals have different abilities these should be welcomed and used appropriately
- no matter how well maintained a team is, problems will arise.

There are no absolute rules to achieving success with the new contract and implementation of the QOF, but hopefully these ideas will help. What is important is that it is not seen as a project to be divided up among a group or the exact division of or carving up of labour, but rather co-ordinated as part of true teamwork.

'Agenda for Change'

Some of the Education quality indicators of the organisational domain of the QOF relate to appraisal. Ultimately, the new contract may not only mean that more is required of staff and more staff time is required, but that staff are given the opportunity to develop new skills to carry out new tasks. This is in line with the 'Agenda for Change' as defined by the Department of Health where the '*Agenda for Change works to harmonise the conditions of service for NHS staff, provide a more transparent system of reward for staff working flexibly, and helps to create the conditions for new kinds of jobs*'.

The pay system associated with the new Agenda for Change applies to all directly employed NHS staff, except very senior managers and those covered by the Doctors' and Dentists' Pay Review Body. This is also to ensure equal pay for work of equal value and so what is referred to as 'Pay Modernisation'.

Further information may be found on the NHS Modernisation Agency website, Agenda for Change, with the following website address: www.modern.nhs.uk/scripts/default.asp?site_id=48.

Perhaps additional staff may also be required. One implication of this is rising staff costs and it is likely that it will be difficult to negotiate an increase in the staff budget which is now included in the Global Sum. When it was a separate item under the 1990 contract, such a negotiation would have been easier.

Appraisal and recognition of achievement and PDPs

The QOF means extra workload and it will expected that the budget for extra staff time or numbers will need to come out of some of the profits gained for providing increased quality of care.

Practical point

Appraisal can praise staff for this as well as setting future targets where bonus payments should be considered with staff if they reach these targets as an incentive. It is important that not just the doctors are seen to benefit financially but that their staff are rewarded for their efforts and loyalty in developing the practice and enhancing quality of care.

A similar argument will apply to the development of in-house services which may be Local or National Enhanced Services, which were discussed in earlier chapters. In relation to the QOF and the other aspects of the new contract, it is important that the team plans and so develops these quality initiatives. This will require both delegation and recognition of achievement as detailed above and regular team meetings.

Staff may be required to learn new skills, e.g., a receptionist learning phlebotomy and extended roles in IT. This can become part of a personal development plan (PDP) for a member of staff. Once learning needs have been identified in relation to the practice professional development plan (PPDP), an appropriate training course should be identified. This approach will enable staff to be more flexible and so may lead to greater job satisfaction and opportunities for members of staff as well as a practice's success in the QOF.

CHAPTER 8

Additional financial issues

The book has so far devoted attention to the Global Sum, enhanced services and the Quality and Outcomes Framework, but there are other important additional issues that should be raised and considered by practices in relation to their income. These are as follows:

- differences between PMS and GMS practices
- seniority payments
- partnerships and the new contract
- premises
- pensions and superannuation
- out-of-hours work
- computers and IT
- dual registration
- goodwill
- PGEA and appraisal
- payments and prolonged study leave (PSL).

Each of these issues will now be discussed in this chapter.

Differences between PMS and GMS practices

PMS or Personal Medical Services will continue under the new contract. PMS practices were in existence before the new GP contract and will have already negotiated a local contract with their PCO. PMS pilots started in 1997 as part of the NHS Plan with the chance to tailor a service to local needs and creatively find better means of flexibly delivering services and so attract more GPs into previously unattractive areas to practise. Therefore the context that patients are seen in will be more appealing and conducive to work in. In relation to recruitment this may mean that the advantages of PMS practices will continue to outweigh those of GMS practices. In addition, prior to the new contract the average earnings of a PMS GP were greater than those of a GMS GP, although with the new contract this gap is likely to become narrower. (Under the new contract GMS practices are sometimes referred to as 'GMS2' practices or new GMS (nGMS) practices.)

This is important as up to 40% of GPs are working in PMS practices. In relation to the new contract some PMS practices may believe that they have the best of both worlds as they can opt out of providing out-of-hours care and what they perceive as restrictive aspects of the QOF as they have a contract that specifically addresses local needs. In addition, PMS practices will retain their present funding, e.g., PMS with growth where a local need has been identified and monies have been made available by the PCO for a salaried doctor or nurse practitioner.

> **Practical point**
> PMS growth monies will not automatically form part of the Global Sum calculations made by PCOs if PMS practices move to GMS after 1 April 2004.

The QOF

In addition to adhering to the QOF, PMS practices should be able to add new domains, alter existing quality indicators or reduce the number of indicators within a domain through negotiation with the PCO. Although PMS practices will be able to run already existing local quality frameworks negotiated under PMS, the total number of quality points available under a locally negotiated framework and the ratio between clinical and non-clinical work (organisational markers) must remain the same as the national GMS framework. This is 550:500 respectively and so a total of 1050 points. Therefore quality targets will need to be agreed between PCOs and PMS practices and be equivalent to the national QOF where possible and practical. Also, most PMS practices will probably opt for the GMS QOF as there will be little time to shape their existing local needs around the tight categories of the quality indicators.

> **Practical point**
> PMS practices will no longer have to give six months notice if they wish to revert to GMS. A time scale can now be negotiated with the local PCO.
>
> Similarly, for practices wishing to change from GMS2 to PMS: there will be no new waves of PMS as GMS practices will be able to apply to go PMS at any time.

A loss of 196 points for PMS practices

Some PMS practice contracts contain monies for chronic disease management and sustained quality allowances. Under the new GMS contract these have been incorporated into the QOF and PMS practices may face a financial deduction so that they are not getting paid 'twice'. This has been estimated as equating roughly with 196 points for 2004/05 and 122 points in 2005/06 when the average value of points increases to £120. These points have since been cut from 196 to 174 and 122.5 to 109 points respectively following a DoH review which indicated an overestimation.

> **Practical point**
> Interestingly for those practices that do differ from the national GMS QOF this may cause them computer software problems as the GP practice software created will be specifically for GMS practices.

Local Enhanced Services

In addition to the Global Sum, there are additional payments for enhanced services and performance in terms of the QOF. PMS practices may change to GMS if monies for local services that they have previously provided face competition from GMS negotiations for Local Enhanced Services. GMS GPs as well as PMS GPs will now have the right to commission services, particularly as part of local clusters. The funding gap between PMS and GMS practices will continue to get smaller.

Practical point

Where income for quality has been included in the PMS budget of a practice this will be deducted and substituted by the QOF income.

Out-of-hours costs

PMS practices will be eligible for increases in finances relating to seniority pay, IT, premises, access funds to improve quality and enhanced services and pensions. However, one area where they may differ with PMS is not the right to opt out of out-of-hours cover, but rather the financial cost of doing so. For an average GMS GP this is likely to be in the region of £6000 (6% of the Global Sum). However, for PMS GPs the calculation is made by taking the registered list and dividing it by the average GMS GP's list and multiplying it by the average cost for GMS GP. This figure could therefore work out as considerably more than £6000.

Seniority payments

New seniority payments were introduced in December 2003 and backdated to April 2003. The payments are based on 'reckonable service' for GP principals who have completed at least two full years in such a post. Reckonable service needs to be of at least eight years in total in the NHS before doctors are eligible for seniority payments. GPs should have been requested by their respective PCOs to produce evidence to establish the reckonable service that they have undertaken. (A GP principal was defined as a practitioner eligible for a basic practice allowance (BPA).)

Overseas doctors will be disadvantaged because of the new rules as 'reckonable service outside the EU' will not count. Under the old contract as defined in the Red Book, the payment was calculated from a doctor's qualifying date. It is therefore based on length of clinical service in the NHS.

To complicate matters, PMS practice GPs can choose to calculate their seniority payments in either of two ways: first, to uplift the whole contract budget by 3.225% which is equivalent to the uplift in GMS fees of 2.85% and their increase in seniority; second, to uplift the whole contract budget by 2.85% and then to add the exact amounts of seniority that would be calculated under the GMS contract.

Seniority payments will vary according to whether a doctor is part-time or is in a job-share, but not if they are in receipt of an inducement payment. Those doctors who have been working as a medical officer in HM forces will need to ask their PCO to seek advice from the Secretary of State as to which period of time can be accepted.

Partnerships and the new contract

One of the big changes of the new contract is that patients are no longer registered with individual GPs, but the practice. Earnings will be paid to practices rather than individuals and this will affect practices who have run 'personal lists' and do not 'pool' all the income. For this reason alone a new practice agreement may be required as the financial structure of practices is changing rather than allowing the doctors to 'move into a partnership at will'. It is also likely that the balances in relation to work in a partnership may change and these need to be acknowledged and discussed so that an appropriate agreement can be negotiated which makes all the partners feel secure in relation to partnership shares.

The implications of the QOF on profits

In relation to additional income from the QOF it may be possible to identify a 'financially under-performing GP', e.g., through the completion of computer templates for the clinical domain of the QOF. Bearing this in mind, who makes judgements about the skill mix in a partnership and the division of profits? These have the potential to become areas of contention. Does a new partnership deed require to take these differences into account? Other issues may arise related to a salaried doctor and a practice where the profits increase under nGMS or the introduction of a non-medical partner, such as a practice manager.

Factors that can affect a partnership agreement

There have been many changes as a result of the new contract which may affect a partnership agreement that mainly reflects the financial structure of a practice. Furthermore, in relation to the PCO, contracts are with the practice rather than individual partners. In January 2004 practices were asked to sign whether to become 'Health Service Bodies' or whether to remain private contractors who can choose to use NHS procedures if they wish as from 1 April 2004. Negotiating rights regarding these two options are to be resolved in due course.

Other changes include:

- Global Sum and provision of essential services
- additional and enhanced services
- the QOF
- recent changes where practices have changed from GMS to PMS.

Further issues where change is presently occurring include:

- leave for maternity, paternity or adoption
- appraisal and revalidation
- prolonged study leave (sabbaticals).

The list is endless and all these issues need to be thought about in advance and provision made for them in the partnership agreement so that they do not come as a surprise to partners. If they are fair and previously negotiated this will ensure a happy partnership rather than one that is constantly in dispute as they did not wish to consider change or to embrace it.

Partnerships at will

It has been estimated by some sources that up to 50% of GPs in the UK do not have an effective partnership deed and have partnerships at will. Establishing a new agreement or updating a partnership deed will inevitably incur legal costs and these could be in the region of £2000. In an ideal world to reduce costs, the GPC of the BMA should have produced a model partnership agreement to accompany the new contract. However, it is likely that an advisory document on partnership agreements will be produced soon, but that it cannot be a model agreement applicable to the great variety of GP practices that exists. It is perhaps an opportunity for practices to discuss where they are now and plan for the future at a time of considerable change to the traditional form of general practice to which many of us have become accustomed. Such changes may already have been made to partnership agreements in PMS practices.

Premises

Primary care is changing rapidly particularly in relation to the new contract. In order to meet the challenges that these changes create in the infrastructure, practice buildings will play a crucial role.

Premises will need to meet three needs:

- patients' expectations
- doctors' aspirations
- the additional services generated by the new contract.

In addition, premises will require to meet defined standards in relation to:

- patients with disability – this includes patients who require wheelchair access or patients with impairment of vision or hearing
- appropriate facilities, e.g., for nappy changing
- adequate lavatory and washing facilities
- waiting areas with enough seating and that ensure confidentiality is maintained
- fixtures, fittings and furniture are in good repair and clean
- provision of adequate lighting, heating and ventilation
- suitably equipped and dedicated treatment room
- facilities for storage and disposal of clinical waste
- fire precautions with safe exits
- security of patient records, prescriptions, associated paperwork and any medications.

These are all important and no one would dispute these needs and standards. However, they require finance and in relation to finance and premises this is a complex area and one that constantly seems to be being revised. This section is intended to give the reader a greater understanding of the background, but if a practice is contemplating development of existing premises or new premises as a result of the new contract, they should talk to their local PCO to find out what is available locally.

Funds for premises

The new contract is moving to a cash-limited fund that has the potential to stifle much-needed developments of premises. Prior to the new contract and development deals signed before 30 September 2003, the funds for premises developments were non-cash-limited (non-discretionary) and held centrally. From 1 April 2004, this has been replaced by a single unified funding stream. This is intended to meet the development needs of all the primary care estate and not just individual general practices and so there is competition. (Primary care estate could include general practices, but may also include community health clinics and walk-in centres.)

The monies for improvements will be allocated to the 28 strategic health authorities (SHAs) for premises growth and each SHA will choose a lead PCO to consider applications for financial assistance. These applications will be considered according to priorities for that area. With a cash-limited fund there is an anxiety that many practices with inadequate premises will not be able to reach the standards that they and their patients would ideally aspire to, particularly to meet the service demands of the new contract. Perhaps an argument that practices need to present to their respective PCOs is that their buildings need to be 'fit for purpose'.

The finance available will be divided up into three areas:

- development of existing premises
- funding for approved schemes prior to 30 September 2003
- annual growth funds.

Annual growth funds will be for strategic service developments, such as new premises, and these will be competitive. One other area of funding that has been developed is that of using public funds from the Treasury which can enable developments under public–private partnerships and these include Local Improvement Finance Trust (LIFT) schemes and the Private Finance Initiative (PFI) respectively. Practices wishing further information on these schemes should talk to the premises development lead at their PCO. There is also guidance available on several websites including the BMA website.

PMS funding will not be directly affected by this new system and so the immediate implications for PMS practices are not the same as GMS practices.

Practical point
When considering an upgrade practices should be considering if they will be prepared to offer extra services, such as enhanced services under the new contract. If they are, then PCOs are more likely to consider their applications.

Cost and notional rents

Under the new contract, premises will continue to receive rent (cost and notional) and rates reimbursement. In addition, premises can still be:

- rented
- purchased
- built by the partnership or a third party.

One change that has come about as a result of the new contract is that practices who are receiving cost rent and then make a capital investment in their premises, e.g., through an extension, will receive a notional rent in addition to the cost rent. This is referred to as an enhanced notional rent factor or 'top up'. This will enable premises development where it is needed and PCOs will prioritise funds to areas of need which are likely to be inner cities and areas of deprivation. Rural areas should be aware that there is a move for some primary care services to be centralised to reduce costs and patients are being increasingly expected to travel rather than have individual services, particularly in rural locations.

Premises: 'fit for purpose'

A further change with the new contract is the guarantee of a minimal sale price for practices in inadequate premises, such as a terrace house, to move to a building that is 'fit for purpose'. This can help with the disposal of properties that might otherwise prove difficult to sell in areas of negative equity.

The systems that surround notional and cost rent will not be directly affected by the new contract. When negotiating a notional rent this will need to be done with the district valuer who is a surveyor as occurred under the 1990 GP contract.

Practical point

If a practice chooses to change to a national rent from a cost rent they will not be allowed to revert to a cost rent.

Service charges

One of the great concerns associated with the new contract relates to service charges incurred on practice premises, for example business rates, water rates and hazardous waste. PCOs will be given almost complete discretion in their approach as to these items and also to cost rent and notional rent. There is no requirement that they have to completely meet the present 100% reimbursements for rates or to increase notional rent in line with any recommendations following review. At a time when PCOs are financially stretched they will need to look to other areas of their budget in order to make the necessary financial savings. Perhaps one area of reassurance is that private income generated using practice premises will continue to be allowed up to 10% of earnings without any penalty being incurred.

Allocation of extra monies to premises development

There seems to be debate as to how much extra money has been allocated by government to development of the premises of the primary care estate. One source has stated that an extra £1.6 billion was being made available nationally by the exchequer to facilitate quality improvement in the 'built environment' of practice premises. However, the need for development of practice premises as a result of the new contract, and the associated clinical work, may require much greater funding. Inevitably, bigger and better premises will be needed, but some sources suggest that many PCOs are facing a shortfall on their premises budgets for the coming year.

Practical point

If practices are finding it difficult to get appropriate premises development considered for funding, they should seek input from their LMC representatives.

PCOs will be required to carry out an audit of their primary care estate. One area of considerable and likely expense is that which relates to the Disability Discrimination Act 1995 and the modernisation of existing premises that may be needed to meet the requirements of the Act. A potential problem that may arise for some practices is whether it is more appropriate for the amalgamation and sharing of premises in the future rather than maintaining individual small practice premises. There also seems to be a political impetus to reduce the number of single-handed practices despite the arguments for the quality of care they provide through the continuity of a personal doctor.

Practical point

For those practices who incur costs relating to possible capital allowances – for example, expenditure on the fabric of the building such as a central heating system – it may be possible to gain a tax refund and advice should be sought from the practice accountant.

Reference

Watkins J (2004) New contract, new premises: new opportunities for development. *The New Generalist.* 2(1): 77.

Pensions and superannuation

A book could be written on this and issues from 'added years' to pensions. This section will limit itself to changes in pensions related to the new contract. With the new contract has come a forecast of a big increase for GP pensions and it is hoped that this will further aid GP recruitment. The difference between the pensions of hospital consultants and GPs is that hospital consultants' pensions are based on their final salary. However, GP pensions are based on their career earnings and they also receive a lump sum on retirement. This is where it becomes complex as in the past under the 1990 contract superannuation was based upon a percentage of an individual GP's income from a GMS practice as follows.

- Most item of service payments were treated as 66% superannuable.
- Target payments, seniority payments and training grants were treated as 100% superannuable.
- Other items, mainly reimbursements, were treated as 0% superannuable, e.g., staff reimbursement.

For PMS practices, the superannuable income was determined by the PCO based on the income for the baseline year (last GMS year) with an annual uplift based on the review body increases.

Changes under the new contract

Under the new contract, as patients are registered with the practice and not individual GPs, superannuation payments will be based on the NHS profits of the practice minus its expenses. So if a practice buys a lot of new equipment or takes on new staff this may result in a possible reduction in superannuation. An estimate of this profit will be made so that an amount can be paid for the employer's contribution (14%) where the notional employer is the PCO and this amount can be deducted from the Global Sum.

In total deductions will be 6% in respect of the employee contribution and 14% employer contribution. Each contractor will be receiving a pre-arranged amount of money to cover their estimated employer contribution costs from the PCO.

> **Practical point**
> At the end of the financial year, the actual superannuable income should be determined by the practice accountant and agreed with the PCO and a balancing adjustment made in respect of contributions. Payment is likely to be made well into the following financial year and practices may need to keep some money set aside to pay this balance. Practices should also request a written monthly statement as proof of payment of superannuation.

Change to retirement age

For GPs 20% of superannuable income is paid to the NHS Pensions Agency and this comprises 6% employee's contributions and 14% as PCO notional employer contributions. With this increase in superannuation, the age required to draw a full pension will be increased from the age of 60 to 65. In addition the earliest age that any GP could retire and draw a pension will rise from 50 to 55 years of age. Unlike the 1990 GP contract practices will have to make payment for both of these contributions and agree amounts with the PCO that will be taken from the practice's Global Sum on a monthly basis.

GPs working for an out-of-hours service will be eligible for superannuation on this income if it is a non-profitmaking organisation. A similar circumstance will arise if a GP works as a clinical assistant at a local hospital NHS trust.

Salaried and locum doctors

Practices will be responsible for employee doctors and their superannuation and it is important to communicate to the PCO regarding such doctors so that the relevant amounts can be deducted from the Global Sum. For those doctors who are in training grades, such as GP registrars, practices should deduct the employee part of superannuation only and the PCO will arrange with the local postgraduate medical education deanery about the employer contributions. For practices who employ locums who are reimbursed by the PCO, the locums may seek the employer contributions of 14% from the PCO as from 1 April 2004. Locums should keep a record of all their NHS work and send their 6% contribution to the appropriate

PCO monthly. The PCO should then add the employer's contribution before sending the payment to the NHS Pensions Agency.

Annual uplift for inflation

Each year of income is increased by a 'dynamising factor' to bring it into line with the current average income of a GP. In other words the longer ago income was earned, the higher this dynamising factor. It is thought that this factor under the new contract may rise by up to 30% over the next three years as it is brought into line with GPs' actual increased earnings and not just inflation and a variety of other economic factors as it was under the 1990 contract to make it the same as the annual pay review. It has been suggested therefore that GPs do not retire before 1 April 2006, as the dynamising factor may not be known until that time and so how an individual GP might benefit from this new arrangement.

Practical point

It is important to ensure that each GP has their income superannuated and it is very important to keep a record of all superannuated income. The NHS Pensions Agency in Fleetwood should be able to provide an individual doctor with their superannuation record on request (NHS Pensions Agency, 200–220, Broadway, Fleetwood, Lancashire FY7 8YS).

The changes of the new contract to pensions are in the way the dynamising factor and superannuable income are calculated as well as the increase to employer's superannuation contributions from 7% to 14%. Also certain income such as premises and drug profits may become superannuable for the first time.

Cap on pensions

There is to be a £1.5 million lifetime cap on each person's pension funds to commence on 1 April 2005 and this has been referred to as 'A' day. This has led some GPs to consider early retirement rather than face a tax of 55% if their pensions and benefits fund exceeds this level. It is thought that the level may rise to £1.8 million over the next four years. However, this issue is complicated by the possible increase in GP earnings under the new contract and that some high-earning GPs could exceed this cap within a short period of two to three years. It would seem good advice that all GPs register their pension plans before the pension rule comes into force as this will exempt them from the cap. GPs may need to seek advice from pension experts or financial advisers regarding this. The reason the government seems to have made this change is that pension payments in the long-term may be unsustainable given increased longevity.

Increase in employer's superannuation contribution and staff pensions

The new contract has brought with it increased funding to compensate for the rise in the employer's superannuation contribution for the employed staff at a GP practice as well as the GPs themselves. The employer's contribution rises this year from 7% to 14%. GPs have previously paid the employee share (6%) and look to the PCO to reimburse the employer share which is now 14%. The 14% employer contribution will be borne by the practice. To compensate for this a 'superannuation premium' based on the 'weighted list' discussed in Chapter 2 will be paid to practices, but the amount is still under negotiation.

Practical point

It should be pointed out that this rise of employer's superannuation contributions to 14% from 1 April 2004 applies to both GPs and their staff. It is important to clarify with the local PCO the superannuation funding for staff, including salaried doctors.

It also needs to be clarified where this additional funding will be paid. If it is paid through the Global Sum it will in effect increase the value of the payment per patient. However, if it becomes part of the correction factor of the MPIG the additional funding may be lost in the years to come as the Carr-Hill formula is recalculated and the correction factor reduced by the amount of the increase that is then given to the Global Sum.

Practical point

This section illustrates how important and complex superannuation and pensions are. It is vital therefore that the practice accountant calculates the year ended net NHS profit figure as soon as possible for the reasons already detailed.

Out-of-hours work

It could be argued that the deciding factor that led to nearly 80% of GPs voting in favour of the new contract was the choice to be able to opt out of out-of-hours cover and so the traditional 24-hour responsibility that GPs have maintained since 1948. There will be many arguments for and against this choice but at a point when daytime general practice is busier than ever many GPs do not feel able to provide out-of-hours cover as well. However, it is recognised that in order to continue provision of out-of-hours cover, PCOs will need to be able to fund this cover which will become their responsibility by the end of 2004. Most GPs will be able to opt out unless they apply late or their PCO declares that there are 'exceptional circumstances' which will prevent them from dropping this responsibility. In addition, this opt-out will include Saturday mornings.

One argument for not opting out are concerns over the quality of the service that will replace the present service in addition to the reduced continuity of care that will result. If the quality of the service is less than the present time this has implications for daytime work of GPs which is likely to increase. It also has implications for the workload of accident and emergency departments. Indirectly this has financial implications as PCOs will need to pick up the cost of increased attendances at accident and emergency departments. Depending on what happens more GPs may volunteer to do shifts on new out-of-hours services run by PCOs to ensure that quality of care for their patients continues. Perhaps the way forward for the future is a more integrated service which is shared by accident and emergency departments, minor injury units and primary care out-of-hours services which pivot around a successful triage system.

It has been estimated that individual GPs in a practice will have an average of £6000 (6% of the Global Sum) a year deducted from their Global Sum if they decide to opt out of out-of-hours cover. Extra money is being made available to PCOs for out-of-hours modernisation over the next three years. It is believed that about half of GPs may offer to do shifts for PCOs providing out-of-hours cover. The remuneration is likely to be much greater than at the present time working for commercial deputising services or GP co-operatives. Also, as previously stated, if the organisation is non-profitmaking such income should be eligible for superannuation.

One further financial implication of changes in out-of-hours cover is for GP co-operatives which are presently owned by local groups of GPs and whether the local PCO will choose them as the out-of-hours provider. In relation to the new contract, this will be one of the most interesting developments as many GP co-operatives and commercial deputising services have taken over a decade to develop their present services and the PCOs have been given a much shorter period of time in comparison.

Computers and IT

In order to maximise income under the new GP contract, practices will need to use computers for patient records with appropriate GP computer software of which there are presently several versions. In relation to the QOF, this has been detailed fully in the previous two chapters. Claims for the quality indicator points of the QOF can only be made if the required patient data has been entered into the computer system using the correct Read codes. It could be argued that appropriate software could take a lot of the stress out of the new GP contract and data entry.

Advantages of computers

For practices who do not use computers or are only using them on a partial basis, this will be a time of considerable change for all members of the practice team and it would be worth seeking advice from the local PCO about equipment and training. Initially this will be daunting to practices that do not use computers or only use them to a limited extent. However, there are many advantages to the use of computers and some of these can be summarised as follows:

- a patient record that is legible
- records that are automatically filed
- summaries that are easily available
- patient information that can be transferred immediately
- integration of records to simplify communication between team members
- a record of all prescribing and an efficient repeat prescribing programme
- a system to recall patients for review
- an excellent method to claim fees from the PCO electronically

- no longer a need to maintain handwritten files and folders or to handwrite letters
- a tool to facilitate audit.

In addition, computers may be used for other tasks in the practice such as collating figures on a spreadsheet, e.g., with the practice accounts.

Change in culture to the use of computers

To be successful under the new GP contract, all members of the practice team need to embrace the use of computers in the workplace. This will involve changing culture and working practice and this needs to be addressed sensitively. As the need for data entry becomes apparent this may be a helpful stimulus to see the advantages of such change. The management of patient information in the NHS is one of the keys to both its efficiency and the quality of care that it can provide and ultimately its success. The notion of a paperless NHS has many advantages, but even if the necessary IT is available it is no use unless practitioners are adequately trained and confident in its use. PCOs will need to work with practices to ensure that the necessary funding is available for training.

An issue that should be considered is that of universal patient record software in primary and secondary care, rather than the present situation of different programs. This may involve practitioners requiring training on several different types of software until a universal package is agreed on.

National Programme for IT (NPfIT)

There have been several recent developments in relation to IT and the NHS that in the future will make it impossible for practices to continue without computer systems. First, it is anticipated that in the near future patients will carry a 'smart' card with their medical records which can be recognised and used in all areas of the NHS, e.g., attending an accident and emergency department. The centralisation of patient data and the ability of the NHS to connect with over 30 000 GPs and other members of the team into a single secure national system is referred to as the 'national data spine'. For a patient this will include details such as health episodes, medications, allergies and much other vital information that is required when a patient is ill. It appears that the contract for the provision of this has been secured with a major service provider. This development is part of the National Care Record Service (NCRS). This change is concurrent with the new GP contract and part of an enormous development that is gathering pace and is referred to as the National Programme for IT (NPfIT).

NPfIT is likely to computerise all aspects of healthcare in the UK over the next ten years and that all communications between every part of the NHS will be electronic. This means that all NHS practitioners will be able to see patient records and associated data when they need to. There are some issues that require to be considered. Perhaps the most important is that most existing GP software will be integrated or replaced and some practices may have to switch to particular brands of software. Issues of what happens to the many practices who are using what might be referred to as 'third-party software' as part of existing IT systems, e.g., for patient appointments, will need to be addressed.

Existing GP software

There is an issue for a universal system and software packages that was alluded to earlier. Until then it is anticipated that there will be a Local Service Provider for each of five regions within England. These will support existing clinical systems software to maintain a working infrastructure for the NPfIT until there is a tested and agreed system to move to. Over the last decade several functional and well-developed software systems have come into being and are being successfully used on a daily basis in practices and it may be difficult to 'better' these systems. The transfer of data to a new system has considerable cost implications for PCOs. On the positive side, the proposed use of centralised servers in data warehouses will be beneficial to many practices as there will be the full-time system administrators available. The issue of increased security of access to information systems cannot be stressed highly enough and methods are being developed to identify the practitioner 'user' who is entitled to have access to this data.

Practical point

Practices wishing to upgrade or change their present computers will need to make a case with their local PCO as all practices are shortly to receive a major upgrade as a result of the NPfIT. However, PCOs will own any of these new systems that they purchase for practices. Maintenance will therefore be met by the PCO. A discussion will take place as to what items are 'core' and what are 'non-core', e.g., flat screens and portable hand-held devices. This is presently being negotiated by the GPC of the BMA.

Training

If there is to be a transition to a universal NHS software, a smooth transition needs to be facilitated and this will involve training and protected time out of practices and is a task that should not be underestimated. Perhaps it is an argument to preserve what we have in general practice until the rest of the NHS can catch up. Even with the present systems that are available, further training is required, not to mention IT support.

Booking patient appointments online and its implications

The second recent development is that GPs will soon be able to book patient appointments in secondary care online, thus considerably improving the existing system. However, such a process takes time, and time that GPs do not have in ten-minute consultations. If this work is then to be taken on by a clerical member of the primary healthcare team, this has implications for increased resources of staff budgets under the Global Sum.

Further developments

There are further developments in the future which relate to the use of computers in practices. These have financial implications not least because of the system and software upgrades that will be required. Many of these are happening concurrently with the new GP contract and are as follows:

- the transmission of laboratory results online (already happening in many areas)
- electronic transmission of prescriptions to pharmacies
- protecting patient confidentiality and complying with the Data Protection Act
- the speed at which electronic data can be transferred and the need by the NHS to use methods such as Broadband.

Funding

With such huge changes in use of IT likely to happen in the near future there is uncertainty over the funding as it is difficult to be specific about the scale of funding that is required. The impact of computers in the consultation can be debated as practitioners spend greater amounts of time inputting data onto computer templates. However, such technology is the only easy way to both record and audit data and so enable GP practices to demonstrate quality of care as required by the new contract.

Under the new contract PCOs will be responsible for helpdesk and IT support services for GP practice computer systems. This responsibility should provide 100% funding for the purchase, maintenance, upgrade and running costs of systems and should be backdated to 1 April 2003. They will also be responsible for the upgrade of systems that are rapidly becoming out of date. Similarly, PCOs will be responsible for ensuring that new systems have the capacity to enable the electronic booking of hospital outpatient appointments.

If this vision is to succeed, similar changes will need to take place in secondary care IT But perhaps the greatest concern of GP practices is the back-up that will be available for this new vision. Why? Previous experience shows that response times are often very slow and when a system is 'down' this prevents the practice from working normally. Similarly, what happens if the system is infected by a virus?

One question that is likely to be asked is who will pay for consumables in a practice such as stationery and printer toner or ink? It is most likely that PCOs will deem these as business expenses and so they will not be covered under any funding agreement.

Practical point

This section hopefully illustrates the many concurrent changes in IT with the new contract. The DoH has commissioned a national QOF Management and Analysis System (QMAS) to handle QOF payments and confirm them to PCOs. Practice computer systems will need to be RFA99-accredited for this to happen. Further details are available on the Primary Care Contracting division of the National Primary and Care Trust Programme: www.natpact.nhs.uk/primarycarecontracting/.

In conclusion, PCOs, rather than practices, will in the future fund the purchase, maintenance, upgrading, running and training costs of GP practice computer (IM&T) systems. Under the 1990 contract many of these were partially reimbursed, rather than fully funded.

Dual registration

Two reasons have been suggested as to why some patients might have 'dual registration'.

1   The DoH document, 'Sustained Innovation through new PMS Arrangements', proposes a pilot scheme for patients to receive specialist PMS care at a designated practice and the rest of their 'essential primary care' from the practice where they are registered.
2   The government's patient choice consultation exercise, 'Building on the Best', proposes that commuters could register with a GP near work as well as one where they live as part of a workplace registration plan.

Understandably these proposals have caused much controversy as they may be very difficult to administer and although a patient would only technically be registered once, they would have an additional but different type of registration.

It might improve management of demand, but may not be practical as overstretched practices where recruitment of doctors is difficult may not be able to meet a further increase in requests for healthcare. It would jeopardise continuity of care and patients may start to seek 'second' opinions from each of the two practices and there would be complications regarding records and the supply of medications. Some sources have suggested that some patients are not worried by continuity of care, but just quick access. This could ultimately mean that patients register with the NHS rather an individual practice.

These issues are going through a process of consultation and whatever the outcome they are likely to have financial implications. For example, it may involve a practice in an increased workload and an equivalent of temporary resident or emergency treatment fees may require to be introduced as happened under the 1990 GP contract.

List closures

Under the new contract if a practice list is officially 'closed' to new patients, that practice may not be able to gain enhanced services funding. If a practice has to forfeit this funding this will have major financial implications for a practice. This is a dilemma for practices who are unable to manage more patients and so a further increase in workload. A process of 'informal closures' would seem fairer as a practice has a right to refuse to take patients onto a practice list as long as it is not discriminatory and that a reasonable written explanation is provided for the decision. However, the refusal can only be temporary if the patient resides in the catchment area, otherwise the practice will be in breach of contract.

Goodwill

When a GP has worked in a practice for a period of time they will have created a 'business' through a growing reputation and the building of good relationships that, as well as providing healthcare, generates an income, which is the basis of this book. This needs to be worked hard at to provide quality care so that patients stay with the practice and do not take their 'custom' elsewhere. It used to be that when a GP resigned or retired they could not sell this work or 'goodwill'. Instead, the remaining partners would expect an incoming doctor or partner to work for a share less than the other partners for a specified period of time until they reached a full share or what is referred to as parity. The other role an incoming doctor might initially adopt was that of 'an assistant with a view', rather than a profit sharing-partner.

It transpires that GPs in England and then possibly Wales, Scotland and Northern Ireland may be permitted to sell the 'goodwill' of a practice as from 1 April 2004. The GPC of the BMA is waiting for further guidance regarding this in relation to established competition law. (At present in the new GMS Contract Framework Document, paragraph 7.21, the sale of goodwill is specifically prohibited.)

Definitions of goodwill

Goodwill may be defined as an estimate of the current and expected profit from the practice In addition to assets such as the premises. On 25 March 2004, the BMA website (www.bma.org.uk) defined goodwill as follows:

> Goodwill can be described as the value over and above tangible assets (for example, premises and equipment) that a business may earn in relation to its undertakings, or which potentially may be earned in the future. It tends to be based on the profitability of a business.

In other words, it is the value or profitability of a business over and above its tangible assets. For GP practices, this can be translated into the 'value' of the patients who regularly use the services of that practice. In countries such as New Zealand this has happened since the formation of the NHS in 1948, but not so with the UK. When the NHS was established in 1948, the government 'compensated' GPs for giving up their right to sell goodwill in order to become part of the NHS. The 'ban' of the sale of goodwill may be partially lifted in England, but this will only apply to non-essential services. The sale of goodwill by all providers (GMS and PMS practices) may therefore apply to:

- additional services
- enhanced services
- out-of-hours services.

However, the ban on the sale of goodwill continues to apply to the provision of essential services and if approved the DoH will review the outcome of this decision in two years. No mention in the GPC letter from the BMA dated 25 March 2004 is made regarding the QOF and the sale of goodwill.

The ban has applied to GP practices, unlike say accountants, as most of the business of a GP practice is 'funded' by the state. In ethical terms the 56-year-old ban has been on the ability to trade in the potential 'value' or 'profitability' of patients. A ban does not apply on private secondary care services.

Why change the ban on goodwill?

The political thinking behind this idea is to make general practice a more popular option for private companies to invest in practices, e.g., to run additional, enhanced or out-of-hours services. These are the areas of the new contract that practices or PCOs may subcontract to the commercial services. This may help to plug gaps in services and perhaps ease workload for practices through new providers, thus increasing the capacity of primary care. The disadvantage is that this may fragment GP services with alternative commercial providers being used and so further loss of the continuity of care. This also has the potential to open the primary care budget to the private sector. Or it may mean that GP partners can use the profits made on non-essential services to employ salaried doctors to run the essential services. With the new contract the obligations on the daily commitment and attendance of a GP at a practice has changed, unlike the terms of service a GP was bound by under the previous 1990 GP contract.

A recent BMA News Review article regarding the sale of goodwill suggested it could lead to primary care services which are less:

- co-ordinated
- integrated
- holistic.

Setting up a limited company in order to 'trade' goodwill

Goodwill can only be traded on services other than essential services as previously defined, e.g., enhanced services or the out-of-hours services. This would necessitate a practice setting up a limited company or separate partnership within a practice to separate additional new services under the new contract from essential services – in other words, two separate entities. Goodwill can be valued according to turnover and profitability. It may be that some GPs who do not opt out of 'out-of-hours' cover may be able to use this as an asset, e.g., selling shares as part of a GP co-operative service. A disadvantage of the sale of goodwill is that younger GPs may not become partners as the cost of 'buying in' to a partnership could be too high and a salaried option with no responsibilities may be their preference.

Goodwill could also be extended to other non-NHS services that GPs undertake as independent contractors, e.g., seeing private patients or being the occupational health doctor to a local company or football team.

Selling goodwill

It is not a guaranteed payment to a GP leaving a practice, but a GP has the potential to gain from their years of service to a practice and so a boost to their pension if they are retiring. However, it is only worth what another doctor is willing to pay for it. In years to come this could be beneficial in a high-earning practice, but at a time of difficulty in recruiting and retaining GPs, it may not be a realistically nego-tiable issue for an incoming doctor who is considering joining a practice where there is below average profitability. Then there may also be a further expense of buying in to their share of the premises. Further guidance on the sale of goodwill is expected from the GPC of the BMA soon and whether this will be permitted as described for non-essential services.

PGEA and appraisal

PGEA (the Postgraduate Education Allowance) has finally ended following its intro-duction with the 1990 GP contract. For many there will be mixed feelings as the culture of collecting points through attendance at PGEA-approved educational meetings has stopped.

Why was PGEA introduced?

One answer might be a stimulus to attend continuing medical education (CME) sessions or courses. In order to claim the PGEA fee GPs had to provide evidence that they were keeping up to date by attending 30 hours of approved CME in the three categories of:

- service management
- disease management
- health promotion.

The PGEA was a valued reimbursement of £2945 for attending the required 30 hours in what was referred to as a PGEA year. Or the allowance could be claimed for an accredited personal development plan (PDP). In 1998 DoH papers on conti-nuing professional development (CPD) suggested a move from the unstructured traditional PGEA continuing education for GPs by transition to the accreditation of PDPs. These plans were accredited by a local GP tutor and a further PDP accredited the following year if the GP produced evidence of their learning after 12 months based on their PDP.

Appraisal and revalidation

During 2003, appraisal became compulsory and a completed 'Form 4' of the official DoH appraisal pro forma provides a summary of the appraisal, together with the agreed action plan and resultant PDP for the forthcoming year. As the year progresses, evidence of learning as a result of implementation of the PDP should also be kept in a portfolio for review at a GP's annual appraisal. In theory, a PDP should be able to be used as a bargaining tool with a PCO for protected learning time and appropriate resources so that the quality of care a GP can provide will be further optimised, e.g., developing the expertise to run a Local Enhanced Service.

Payment for CPD, the Global Sum and the new GP contract

The monies for PGEA and appraisal are now to be included within the Global Sum, which is a figure calculated on many of the item of service fees paid to GPs under the previous contract, as detailed in Chapter 2. This has implications for the future of CPD for GPs as the derivation of this fee may be difficult to identify. Therefore, specifically 'ringfencing' it for training could become blurred unlike the distinct PGEA allowance.

In relation to learning needs and defining learning objectives, PDPs are likely to relate much more to service needs such as chronic disease management and the QOF of the new contract. Thus, the culture of lunchtime and evening meetings may rapidly diminish and disappear as attendance dwindles through reduced demand and changing learning needs and styles.

CPD and the GMC

In paragraph 10 of the GMC publication, *Good Medical Practice (GMP)*, doctors are informed that they are responsible for keeping themselves up to date in all areas of their practice (www.gmc-uk.org). Revalidation (which is still to be finally agreed upon) will mean that doctors will need to be able to demonstrate that they are up to date and fit to practise medicine.

> *You must keep your knowledge and skills up to date throughout your working life. In particular, you should take part regularly in educational activities which maintain and further develop your competence and performance (GMP, September 2001).*

The outstanding PGEA payment from the 1990 GMS contract

It is my understanding regarding this issue that it should be possible to claim a fee of £2945 for PGEA activity that finished on 31 March 2004. GPs may wish to contact their local PCO for clarification. Why?

The PGEA payments most GPs have been receiving until 31 March 2004 were for the previous year's PGEA claim (from 1 April 2002 to 31 March 2003). Individual 'PGEA years' vary for GPs, but the majority are April to March. PGEA claims submitted just after 31 March 2003 for the PGEA year: 1 April 2002 to 31 March 2003 were paid quarterly in arrears until 31 March 2004.

The new contract Global Sum payment is prospective for ongoing PGEA/CPD from 1 April 2004. The period that GPs may perceive that they require reimbursement for is retrospective under the 1990 GP contract for 1 April 2003 to 31 March 2004. It is important to contact PCOs for claim forms if GPs believe that they may be eligible. Discussion with their LMC may also help to clarify this issue. See the Appendix for further details.

Payments and prolonged study leave (PSL)

Prolonged study leave (PSL) was funded under the NHS by the previous 1990 GP contract, but approval and finance came directly from the Department of Health. Now approval and finance will come from budgets devolved to the PCOs. Furthermore, any doctor who is on a Medical Performers list of primary medical services under a GMS contract may be entitled to apply for PSL.

PSL is to enable GPs to pursue an academic or specialist interest that will be of benefit to their patients, practices and the NHS as a whole. This might be developing the skills to become a GPwSI by gaining a new clinical expertise or studying for a masters degree in a medically related subject or undertaking primary care research.

Step-by-step guide

The Department of Postgraduate General Practice Education of the London Postgraduate Deanery provides a very helpful website with a step-by-step guide to applying for PSL. This may be found at: www.londondeanery.ac.uk/gp/.

These are some of the important steps referred to:

1   Decide why you want PSL.
2   If you are in a GMS practice, contact your Director of Postgraduate General Practice Education (DPGPE) at the local Postgraduate Deanery for an application pack who will hopefully approve your application and recommend it to the PCO. If you are in a PMS practice, your application is currently handled completely by the PCO, with advice usually requested by the PCO from the Deanery.
3   The PCO have to agree to provide funding if a GP is to be granted PSL.
4   Agree the arrangement with your practice including locum cover.
5. Indicate the length of the PSL which can be from 10 weeks to 12 months, full-time or part-time over a longer period of time, e.g., perhaps two sessions a week for three years.
6   Obtain letters of support from the input of any academics involved, your supervisor/mentor/appraiser, your PCO and most important your practice.
7   On your application, give a detailed background including a review of any relevant literature and how it will form part of your PDP.
8   A PSL administrator should be nominated by PCOs to deal with your application.
9   If your application is approved and funding is available from the PCO, it is expected that a report of 3000–5000 words will be provided once PSL has been completed summarising the work undertaken.

Practicalities

If study leave is approved and finance is available, the contractor (the practice) will be entitled to two payments:

a   an educational allowance
b   a locum allowance.

Before finally going ahead with PSL it is important to calculate how much money there will be available for the purposes of, e.g., going on a course as the individual GP using the educational allowance and employing a locum through the locum allowance. In other words, will this arrangement work financially?

Currently the fees are:

- an educational allowance of £129.50 a week
- a contribution up to £948.33 per week towards the cost of employing a locum.

This figure will differ if the GP concerned on PSL is part-time.

Funding

In a short article on the subject Dr Bill Irish writes:

> *The potential problem that many of us foresee, however, is that primary care organisations don't have a ring fenced fund for PSL, and applications may well be considered against other competing funding for educational and clinical needs. It remains to be seen whether PSL will survive in this climate.*

(Irish B (2004) Will prolonged study leave still be possible under the new general practitioner contract? [The Advice Zone] *BMJ* Career Focus. **328:** s112.)

CHAPTER 9

Summary

It is intended that this book should be both a guide and a source of reference for GPs and their practice managers regarding the new contract and its implications for the practice income and how this may be optimised. Inevitably when the book goes into print developments will have taken place as the GPC of the BMA seek to interpret areas of the new contract that require clarification. Similarly, PCOs will also make interpretations in relation to each individual locality. This is an opportunity to write notes beside the text so that the book continues to be a handy reference.

I am keen to receive feedback and to be educated in areas where it is perceived that there are possible misinterpretations and so errors. This can be done through email: rcharlton@doctors.org.uk

There will also be areas in which the reader requires further information and I would refer such enquiries to the BMA website (www.bma.org.uk) and their publications regularly referred to as the two 'Blue Books'.

- *New GMS Contract 2003: Investing in General Practice*
- *New GMS Contract 2003: Investing in General Practice. Supporting Documentation.*

One area of imminent potential development and change relates to enhanced services detailed in Chapters 3, 4 and 5. LMCs are pressing PCOs locally and the DoH nationally to define exactly what are 'core' or 'essential' services and that practices are rewarded for additional services such as the NES for Minor Injuries or the development of appropriate LESs.

The following section is a summary of the book in relation to a potential practice's income.

Breakdown of a practice's income

Payments under the previous 1990 GP contract have been mapped to income streams under the new GP contract. Income to practices from 1 April 2004 will be from the following sources:

- Global Sum (and MPIG as appropriate)
- Enhanced services
- Quality and Outcomes Framework

Further income will arise from:

- PCO-administered funds including seniority payments
- premises, e.g., notional rent
- IT relating to practice computers
- dispensing.

Other income may arise as a result of:

- training and teaching
- prescribing incentives and other local PCO initiatives.

Further pensionable income will arise from increased employer superannuation contributions and the dynamising factor referred to in Chapter 8.

Income will continue to arise from private work and also potentially from 'goodwill' as discussed previously.

What might payment schedules from a PCO look like?

From 1 April 2004 a payment schedule might look like the following:

- Global Sum with MPIG factor if indicated
- details of superannuation contributions
- a twelfth of agreed enhanced service payments
- a twelfth of aspiration payments under the QOF.

In addition there should be payments for:

- premises
- seniority
- training (e.g., of the GP registrars if this is being undertaken)
- dispensing
- agreed locum cover
- other.

Keys to success under the new contract

1   To gain an understanding of the new GP contract, which is the aim of this book, and how the new contract differs from the 1990 GP contract and changes that need to be made in a GP practice as a result. In NHS 'speak' this might be referred to as strategic planning.

2   Use the computer for every activity in the practice as without its full use and potential the practice will lose income. Where possible Read code entries.

3   Involve the practice team and where people excel, then consider introducing a bonus scheme. It is important that the team members' morale is maintained and that they are valued for their many contributions. The doctors will not be able to do all the additional work that will be generated by the new contract.

4   A happy partnership of doctors is where they communicate regularly, share out the increased workload and agree on appropriate delegation to make use of the individual skills of team members.

5   For GPs not to lose sight of their two key 'specialist' areas which are traditional general practice but difficult to measure objectively. Nevertheless they are two areas where our patients appreciate the quality of care that they result in: first, the continuity of care provided by a trusted personal 'family' doctor; and second, working as generalists knowing our limitations, where to refer for specialist input and when.

Appendix

There are elements of the 1990 GMS contract that should, in the author's interpretation, continue as they are paid in arrears for work undertaken prior to 1 April 2004. Under the 1990 GMS contract the old regulations allowed for claims to be submitted for up to six years. However, the limit for submitting these claims may be reduced to six months at a PCO's discretion.

Income from the '1990 contract' should therefore not stop on 1 April 2004. Some of it should continue as many of the payments are in arrears and practice managers should ensure that these continue to be paid or have been settled by 1 April 2004. Individual practices will need to discuss and negotiate such potential claims with their local PCO. If a practice is in doubt they should seek advice from their LMC or the GPC of the BMA.

The following areas relate to the previous 1990 GMS contract.

Item of service fees

Item of service fees that should have been claimed by 1 April 2004 include:

- maternity where there are fees for antenatal care up to 16 weeks, 30 weeks, prior to birth, confinement and postnatal care
- temporary resident
- immediately necessary treatment
- emergency treatment
- arrest of dental haemorrhage
- night visit
- vaccinations/immunisations.

Fees that are paid three months in arrears

GPs' fees under the 1990 GMS contract should have been paid three months in arrears for the following work undertaken in the quarter prior to 1 April 2004. These were as follows:

Payment	Period for which payment is due
Basic practice allowances	For the quarter prior to 1 April 2004
Capitation fees	For the quarter prior to 1 April 2004
Out-of-hours quarterly allowance	For the quarter prior to 1 April 2004
Minor surgery fee for five procedures	For the quarter prior to 1 April 2004
Child health surveillance	For the quarter prior to 1 April 2004

(Health promotion and chronic disease management)	
Health promotion	For the quarter prior to 01.04.04
Diabetes management	For the quarter prior to 01.04.04
Asthma management	For the quarter prior to 01.04.04

Quarterly out-of-hours payments should continue until PCOs take over out-of-hours cover for those practices wishing to opt out of out-of-hours cover from 1 January 2005.

Practical point

While practices are waiting for out-of-hours cover to be implemented, they should ensure that the necessary out-of-hours payments continue and whether or not they have been itemised in the Global Sum.

There are some payments which are payable for work that was done prior to 1 April 2004 and it therefore seems logical to assume that they should continue. This should be negotiated with the local PCO for payment on 30 June 2004 and beyond as follows.

Fees that are paid 12 months in arrears

1   Contraception fees were paid quarterly for 12 months for any person renewing an FP1001 claim within the 12 months preceding 1 April 2004.
2   New patient registration fees were paid for patients who registered at a practice and received a 'new patient medical' within three months of their registration. However, if an adequate reason could be provided as to why this was not possible, but that the 'new patient medical' was still conducted within 12 months of their registration, then the fee could still be claimed.
3   PGEA: if a GP's PGEA year finishes on 31 March 2004 and certification is produced for 30 hours of accredited postgraduate education then payment is due quarterly on 30 June 2004, 30 September 2004, 31 December 2004, 31 March 2005 for the previous 12 months PGEA claim. If a GP's PGEA year finishes at a time other than 31 March 2004, then they should be paid pro rata.

Target payments

This is where the situation becomes complex. If a practice looks at previous payments they will discover that payments should be as follows.

Target payment	Due date for target payment
Childhood immunisation	1 April 2004 for immunisation status at 1 October 2003
Childhood immunisation	1 July 2004 for immunisation status at 1 February 2004
Childhood immunisation	1 October 2004 for immunisation status at 1 May 2004 pro rata

Preschool booster	1 April 2004 for immunisation status at 1 October 2003
Preschool booster	1 July 2004 for immunisation status at 1 February 2004
Preschool booster	1 October 2004 for immunisation status at 1 May 2004 pro rata

However, after the 30 June payment, payment should be made through the Directed Enhanced Service for childhood immunisations and preschool boosters as discussed in Chapter 3.

Target payment	*Due date for target payment*
Cervical cytology	1 April 2004 for target attainment on 1 October 2003
Cervical cytology	1 July 2004 for target attainment on 1 February 2004
Cervical cytology	1 October 2004 for target attainment on 1 May 2004 pro rata

However, it may be argued that further payments are partially covered on the additional services domain of the quality indicators of the Quality and Outcomes Framework of the new contract discussed in Chapter 7.

Area of debate

Financial claims under the previous 1990 contract as detailed above are an area of debate and are being discussed by the GPC of the BMA. The above information and suggestions are the interpretations of the author and it is anticipated that the GPC will provide further advice to GP practices in due course. If a practice believes that they may be eligible to make these claims, they should discuss the matter further with their PCO. If they are unhappy with the outcome, they should talk to their LMC or the GPC of the BMA for further advice.

Glossary

Adjusted Disease Prevalence Factor (ADPF)
Angiotensin converting enzyme (ACE) inhibitor
Angiotension II antagonist (A2)
Body mass index (BMI)
British Medical Association (BMA)
British Thoracic Society (BTS)
Cerebrovascular accidents (CVA) – stroke
Chronic obstructive pulmonary disease (COPD)
Computerised (Axial) Tomography (CT) scan
Continuing professional development (CPD)
Contractor Population Index (CPI)
Coronary heart disease (CHD)
Department of Health (DoH)
Diploma of the Royal College of Gynaecologists (DRCOG)
Directed Enhanced Services (DES)
Echocardiogram (ECHO)
Exercise tolerance testing (ETT)
General Medical Services (GMS)
General Practitioners Committee (GPC)
Global Sum Equivalent (GSE)
Glycosylated haemoglobin (HbA1c)
Gonadotrophin releasing hormone (GnRH)
GPs with a Special Interest (GPswSI)
Health Care Assistant (HCA)
International Normalised Ratio (INR)
Intra-uterine contraceptive device (IUCD)
Left ventricular dysfunction (LVD) - heart failure
Local Enhanced Services (LES)
Local Medical Committee (LMC)
Magnetic Resonance Imaging (MRI) scan
Measles, mumps and rubella (MMR)
Minimum Practice Income Guarantee (MPIG)
Minor Injuries Service (MIS)
Myocardial infarction (MI)
National Enhanced Services (NES)
National Health Service (NHS)
National Institute for Clinical Excellence (NICE)
National Primary Care Development Team (NPDT)
National Programme for IT (NPfIT)
National Service Framework (NSF)
Near-patient testing (NPT)
Patient-Participation Group (PPG)

Personal development plan (PDP)
Personal Medical Services (PMS)
Planning and Priorities Framework (PPF)
PRImary Care Clinical Effectiveness (PRICCE) scheme
Primary care organisation (PCO)
Primary care trust (PCT)
Primary healthcare team (PHCT)
Prolonged study leave (PSL)
Prostate specific antigen (PSA)
Quality and Outcomes Framework (QOF)
QOF Management and Analysis System (QMAS)
Quality Information Preparation Payment (QuIPP)
Quality Preparation Payment (QPP)
Scottish Intercollegiate Guidelines Network (SIGN)
Sexually transmitted infection (STI)
Strategic health authority (SHA)
Thyroid function tests (TFTs)
Thyroid stimulating hormone (TSH)
Transient ischaemic attack (TIA)

Index